Dr Peter Atherton

D0774067

Aloe Vera

The Medicine Plant

'You ask me what were the secret forces which sustained me during my long fasts. Well, it was my unshakable faith in God, my simple and frugal life style, and the aloe, whose benefits I discovered upon my arrival in South Africa at the end of the 19th century'.

Mahatma Gandhi
(in a letter to his biographer Romain Rolland)

© KPM Co.
1st edition 2006

Author: Dr Peter Atherton
Published by: KPM Co.
Printed and bound by: Pergamos-Adam Editions

ISBN: 0-9540896-1-8

Contents

Author's Note

This handbook is designed for educational purposes only and does not endorse any particular brand or type of Aloe Vera product.

Dr Atherton regrets that he is unable to enter directly into any correspondence regarding his opinion on the use of Aloe Vera in particular case studies.

Acknowledgements

I would like to thank all those people who helped me to produce my first book on Aloe Vera, 'The Essential Aloe Vera', on which this, the second book, is based; in particular, my wife Ellen, Glenda Goodwin, Tamsin Wright-Carpenter, Pam Richardson and Nick Hutchins.

I must reserve a special mention for Rosalynd Skinner, without whose help I could not have succeeded in making the various changes, incorporating the new ideas necessary to change the design, style and content, which makes this book so different from the first. Her critical appraisal and textual input has enabled me to present a work that is hopefully intelligible to non-medical as well as the scientific community who both wish not only to use Aloe Vera, but to understand its actions.

I would also like to thank David Urch, a veterinary surgeon, for allowing me to use extracts from his book 'Aloe Vera-Nature's Gift'.

To Ellen

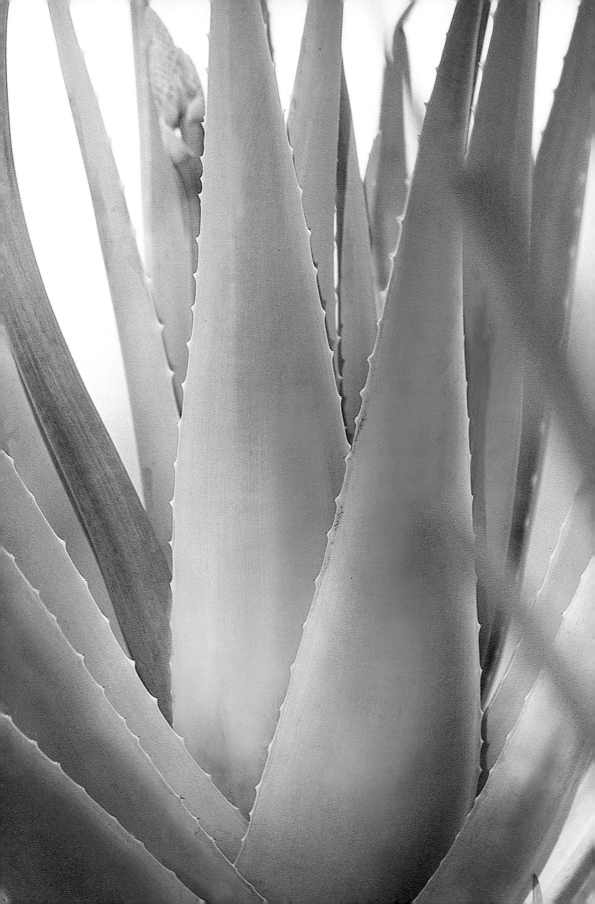

Foreword

Despite decades of scientific research, it remains true that for a wide range of illnesses conventional medicine is of limited effectiveness. It is therefore no surprise that many patients, particulary those suffering from disease which is chronic in the sense of long-lasting, turn to complementary or alternative medical remedies. One of the most widely used of these approaches is herbal therapy, of which Aloe Vera is a prominent example.

As Peter Atherton indicates in this book, Aloe Vera has been used for thousands of years, in several different cultures, as a therapy for a variety of different conditions. There is a wealth of anecdotal evidence suggesting that it is effective, and test-tube experiments have shown that components of Aloe Vera have some actions which could be useful clinically.

Unfortunately, however, reports by individuals of the apparent effectiveness in themselves of a herbal (or other) therapy, cannot prove that the preparation will necessarily work in a population of patients with the same disease. For example, the apparent benefit in a individual instance may be due to a placebo effect or to spontaneous improvement of the illness. Furthermore, people who fail to gain benefit from the treatment will usually not bother to report that it did not work. This means that clinical trials need to be undertaken in which the effectiveness and safety of the herbal remedy are compared, in a group of patients with a particular illness, with those of a matching placebo, or conventional treatment, in a similar group of subjects.

With the help of Peter Atherton, we conducted such a study in patients with ulcerative colitis, a chronic inflammatory diarrhoeal disease, and found evidence that Aloe Vera gel does indeed perform better than placebo when given for six weeks. There is a clear need for more such studies not only in inflammatory bowel disease, but also in wide spectrum of other settings in which Aloe Vera is used.

This book will, I hope, not only interest patients and their therapists in the potential value of aloe vera gel, but also stimulate clinicians to undertake further research to confirm or refute claims of its therapeutic efficacy. If you are a patient thinking of using Aloe Vera, you will find a wealth of fascinating information here. As a 'conventional' doctor myself, I would advise you to discuss any plans you have to use Aloe Vera with your GP or specialist, not least because some herbal therapies can interact with, and alter the effectiveness and safety of other drugs. Meanwhile, enjoy what is written here, and encourage your doctors to push for further scientific evaluation of the potential clinical role of aloe vera gel and other herbal preparations.

D S Rampton
Professor of Clinical Gastroenterology
Barts and The London,
NHS Trust

April 2005

Introduction

"Aloe what? Yes, I think I've heard of that – the stuff they put in cosmetics."

This was the essence of a conversation I had with a patient ten years ago.

She was the mother of a little boy with eczema, whose problem had apparently 'miraculously' completely cleared up after applying a creme containing aloe vera gel and Bee Propolis, a weird – as I thought at the time - sort of antibiotic extracted from bee hives.

The meeting with the mother of that small boy was not only to change my attitude to Aloe Vera, but also to herbal, nutritional and complementary medicine in general. It also changed my approach to the practice of medicine and thus my life.

At the time, however, I was irritated by the mother's remarks. I was also very sceptical when she urged me to try the creme, maybe because it had succeeded where all my moisturisers and steroid cremes had failed. Eczema, of course, is known to naturally wax and wane, so it had to be coincidental, or had it?

At that point, I had been a General Practitioner for 25 years and a strictly conventional one at that. I left it to my partners to indulge in fringe medicine such as acupuncture, homeopathy, applied kinesiology and nutritional medicine.

However, this patient was also a friend and so it was not long before we met again. Inevitably, the subject of Aloe Vera resurfaced. Now, I was being invited to drink it as well as apply it. The more uses she mentioned, the more I switched off and the more resistant I became. However, I knew she wouldn't stop pestering me until I did something. So, beating a hasty retreat, I promised to read the company literature she had given me.

As I expected, the company which produced the product was biased. However, there was something about the herb's history that captured my attention. There were references to Alexander the Great, Cleopatra and Nefertiti, no doubt mythical associations, but ones which nevertheless prompted me to start asking questions. At my request, the secretary of my local post-graduate medical centre began to dig out anything she could find on Aloe Vera.

The result was more than 40 papers from all over the world. Admittedly, some were from fairly dubious sources but, with only one exception, they all waxed lyrical about Aloe Vera. Such a high incidence of enthusiasm and consensus is most unusual in medical papers.

One paper in particular, from the Acne Research Institute (ARI) of California, published in the Journal of Dermatological Surgery on post dermabrasion wound healing, was to commit me to using Aloe Vera myself, as well as in my practice. Due to the fact that my favourite aspect of general practice was skin disease and because the paper was an extremely interesting one, my imagination was fired.

Dermabrasion is a very aggressive way of treating badly scarred skin following the ravages of facial acne. It literally shaves off the epidermis, or skin surface, leaving the raw area of the dermis to heal and regenerate a smoother epidermal layer. This is fine if the healing is swift and it does not become infected. However, it's a risky process and, in the worst cases, can result in further disfigurement.

British medicine is generally more conservative than it is in the USA, so dermabrasion is only rarely performed in the UK. However, during the ARI experiment in California, when aloe vera gel was added to their standard mixture, they found that the side of the face which was treated with aloe vera gel healed consistently 25%-30% faster than the side which had received the regular dressing. The paper concluded by stating:

"The cause of the accelerated healing is not known."

That did it for me. I had to know more about this unusual plant. Ten years later, I'm still excited about its potential and I'm still learning.

As a direct consequence of using Aloe Vera myself, in my family and in my practice, I made the decision to try and research its medicinal properties in depth. By chance, I discovered that any long standing GP could apply for prolonged study leave for up to a year and be subsidised by the National Health Service. Once I had the endorsement of my regional Post Graduate Dean and two referees, I needed to make a case for a research project that would not only promote my own professional growth, but that would also benefit National Health Service patients, so I chose as my subject 'the medicinal qualities of Aloe Vera'.

I doubt that my application would have been successful but for a singular stroke of luck. When I telephoned the Department of Health to check that my application had been received, I was informed by the young man who was responsible for rubber-stamping the document that he had only been in the job a week and wasn't too familiar with the process. Well, I quickly enlightened him about the need for a speedy assessment in order to arrange locums and reorganise my practice. By the time I'd put the receiver down, the application had been stamped, the business had been resolved and I was already planning my sabbatical year.

In a subsequent and fortunate encounter with the Clinical Professor of Dermatology at Oxford, it was suggested that I could also apply for a visiting research fellowship at Green College, Oxford. This meant that I would be able to carry out my research in the Department of Dermatology and work with the Oxford Institute of Wound Healing. I would also have a desk in the visitors' room, which I would share with, amongst others, Dr Gerry Bodecker, Chairman of the Global Initiative for Traditional Systems of Health, or GIFTS of Health as it is more commonly known.

I was soon granted my fellowship and thus began a fruitful and enjoyable association with a group of talented people. I was also able to focus at last on my main aims, to seek out and evaluate international literature written on every aspect of Aloe Vera and to investigate aloe's wound healing properties.

Having read this book, I also hope that more people will have a greater understanding of the properties and uses of Aloe Vera; that they can begin to see for themselves the benefits to be obtained, particularly in areas where conventional medicine may have failed them.

I am certainly not discouraging the acceptance of a conventional approach, however, whilst I do believe that Aloe Vera has a complementary role to play in the management of a number of conditions, it is not just for treating the sick. Healthy people can benefit enormously from its superb qualities, all of which I will discuss.

I hope you will benefit, as I have, from a plant which has been known by many different names in its long history, the Medicine Plant and Potted Physician being just two.

In the ten years since I began studying Aloe Vera, from being almost unheard of in the UK, it has now become an accepted additive to a wide variety of products, from shampoos and moisturisers, to aftershaves and lipsticks, as well as to babies nappies, women's tights and latex protective examination gloves.

Why have all these companies jumped on the aloe bandwagon? Maybe it's because they realise that by adding Aloe Vera they will help to improve the condition of the user's skin through aloe's soothing and moisturising effects, as well as utilising aloe's anti-microbial action. The problem is that although all these companies are keen to put 'Aloe Vera' on the label, they don't usually add enough to the product, so it tends to have little effect. They are actually using 'Aloe Vera' as an advertising gimmick to sell the product. For it to work effectively, a product almost needs to have Aloe Vera as its main ingredient, not just as a minor additive.

May, 2006   Dr Peter Atherton

A Herbal History

The Precursor of Modern Pharmacology

'Excellent herbs had our fathers of old –
excellent herbs to ease their pain'.

Rudyard Kipling: 'Our Fathers of Old'

The medicinal use of herbs is said to be as old as mankind and, until the 18th century, it was the usual form of medical treatment in the west. Today, the value of herbs in the diet and herbs as health remedies are being rediscovered, as people increasingly question the unacceptable side effects of many pharmaceutical drugs.

Herbs also have the distinct advantage of causing very few, if any, side effects providing they are used correctly. Furthermore, there are specific conditions, such as certain forms of eczema, which have responded well to herbal remedies when orthodox medical treatment has failed.

Today the World Health Organisation estimates that, worldwide, herbalism is three to four times more commonly practised than conventional medicine. We are constantly reminded of the influence that folklore has had on medicine over thousands of years, as well as the plants that have provided us with powerful, and sometimes notorious drugs such as heroin from opium poppies; the heart drug, digitalis, from foxgloves; ergot from rye, used to treat migraine; and aspirin from willow bark, to name just a few. Today over 70% of the British Pharmacopaeia originates from herbs, with 121 commonly used prescription drugs owing their origins to 95 different plants.

The difference between orthodox and herbal medicine is that herbalists support the notion of using the 'whole' plant, since they believe that plants are complex and contain many synergistic ingredients that work together to make the plant a potent form of natural medicine, rather than extracting the prime ingredient.

The efficacy of many plants is now being confirmed by modern scientific trials and tests. Mounting evidence now supports the healing power of plants, as researchers compare the safety and efficacy of natural remedies with their chemical counterparts, such as St John's Wort for depression and Saw Palmetto for prostate problems. This has resulted in numerous scientific studies and research papers appearing in highly regarded scientific journals worldwide, including the Lancet and the British Medical Journal.

However, although research continues to investigate the uses of new plants, many doctors and scientists still do not acknowledge that herbs have the power to heal. They prefer to rely on the familiar pharmaceutical drugs in their armoury, despite the fact that our knowledge of herbs can be traced back to Ancient Egypt, where priests routinely and successfully practised herbal medicine.

Primitive tribes still use their early knowledge of plants and their healing properties, passed down through generations over thousands of years. In many early civilizations, food and medicine were inextricably linked, Hippocrates said:

'let medicine be your food and food be your medicine',

and many plants were eaten specifically for their health-giving value. According to historical documents, the Egyptian pyramids were built partly on the strength of garlic. The slave labourers were apparently given a daily ration of garlic to ward off the virulent fevers and infections that were rife at the time. It was at this time that the first herbals, books that describe herbs, and there culinary and medicinal properties, started to be written.

In Europe, from the Dark Ages to medieval times, herbals were painstakingly hand-copied in the monasteries, which had their own physic gardens for growing herbs to treat both inmates and the local community, and in rural Britain, particularly in the west and Wales, the Druids are believed to have had an oral tradition of herbalism.

In the 15th century, the advent of the printing press enabled herbal wisdom to be disseminated more easily with the compilation and publication of herbals. Apothecary shops – the first chemists - were set up, the most famous of these by British herbalist Nicholas Culpeper (1616-54). His most famous herbal, 'The English Physician Enlarged' (1649), is still in print.

Another well-known English herbalist and 'dealer in leeches' was Henry Potter, who set up in London in 1812 and was soon firmly established. By this time, a vast amount of traditional lore on the medicinal use of herbs had been amassed, not just from Britain and Europe, but also from the Middle East, Asia and America. The opening up of trade routes and England's development as a seafaring nation increased this influx of eagerly received information. Potter's name, like Culpeper's, lives on in his much-thumbed herbal, 'Potters Cyclopaedia of Botanical Drugs and Preparations'.

However, despite the popularity of Culpeper, Potter and others of their ilk, the advances of science did not bode well for the herbal fraternity. The power of scientifically inspired medicine gradually sent herbal medicine into a decline, although it continued to be the treatment of choice and necessity in the countryside. In 1864 a group of herbalists, including several who trained in the USA, founded the National Association (now Institute) of Medical Herbalists, a training and standards organisation.

Until well into the 20th century, the Institute firmly resisted the attempts of orthodox medical people to have herbal medicine banned, and public sympathy was largely with the herbalists, thus helping them stay in business. In the 21st century public interest is once again on the increase.

To emphasise its growing importance, the current health minister of the day was recently asked to compile a report on complementary and alternative medicine (CAM) after a lay consultation period. Its purpose was to define the important aspects of the different branches of alternative and complementary medicine, including medical herbalism, as well as to examine the ways in which CAM members can be regulated.

ALOE VERA in History

'Within the infant rind of this weak flower
poison hath residence and medicine power'.

Wm Shakespeare: Romeo and Juliet

Aloe Vera is one of nature's greatest gifts and one of its many eponyms, The Medicine Plant, is a fitting one.

Since earliest times, Aloe Vera has occupied a prominent place in the medicinal folklore of various cultures. According to ancient texts, Nefertiti, Cleopatra and Alexander the Great were all familiar with this small, compact member of the lily family, although several of the stories might have suffered from embellishment over the centuries.

Aloe has also been considered a lucky plant in some cultures, for example in Africa where it was thought to attract good fortune and repel evil; clumps of Aloe Vera were hung above doorways of new homes as a symbol of hope and good fortune by the inhabitants.

In Mexico, potted Aloe Vera plants were placed close to the front doors of houses to ensure that anyone who passed through would have only good intentions. In some countries Aloe Vera plants are wrapped in paper and given to newlyweds without the benefit of planting or watering. If the plant thrives, the couple is supposed to have good luck. If not, the opposite is implied.

The name Aloe Vera, or True Aloe, is thought to derive from the Arabic word alloeh, Syrian alwai, or Hebrew halal, meaning a 'shining, bitter substance' hence the old laxative remedy Bitter Aloes, still listed in the US Pharmacopea today.

German Egyptologist, George Ebers (1837-1898) acquired an ancient papyrus, now called the Ebers Papyrus, dating from the reign of the Pharaoh Amen-Hotep in 1552 BC. This ancient medical treatise listing the use of plant materials as cosmetics and drugs, including Aloes, was discovered between the knees of a mummy excavated near Thebes in 1858. It demonstrates the use of Aloe Vera during the previous 2,000 years and lists 12 different formulae for Aloe Vera preparations.

Most of our knowledge and use of herbs can be traced back to the ancient

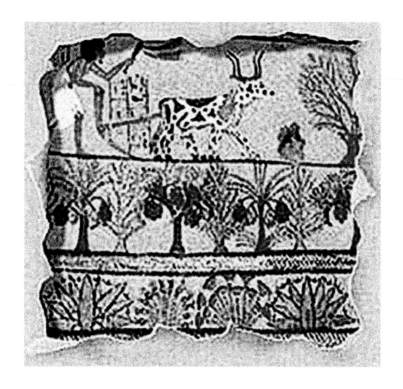

Egyptians, whose priests were also herbal practitioners. The virtues of the plant have also been recorded by other great civilisations, from those of Persia, the Middle East and China, to Greece and Italy in Europe, as well as in India and the African continent. As their armies conquered the then known world, military doctors took the plants and knowledge of their uses with them, gaining new skills as they travelled. To this day, herbs play a vital part in health-care in China, where there are numerous schools of herbal medicine, as well as herbal dispensaries in most hospitals.

During the time of Jesus Christ, important thinkers such as Celsius, through to the Roman physician, Pliny the Elder, and the Greek, Dioscorides, all supported the therapeutic importance of Aloe Vera. Galen, the father of modern medicine, and the first physician to describe how the heart and circulation worked, is also known to have used it in his work.

According to the ancient Indian system of Ayurvedic medicine used in India and now popular in the west, Aloe Vera, or Kumari, is considered one of the most valuable Ayurvedic plants. It has been used to treat a variety of ailments, most commonly bowel disorders such as colic, constipation, diarrhoea and colitis; and skin problems such as eczema, dry skin, itching, burns and cuts.

According to an English translation by John Goodyear in 1655 of Dioscorides' De Materia Medica, written in AD70-90, the bitter-tasting, strongly-scented aloe liquid had

'the power of binding or procuring sleep, of drying, of thickening bodies, and loosening of ye belly and of cleansing ye stomach'. It also 'stops ye spitting of blood and cleanseth ye icterus (liver)'.

As if that weren't enough, this wondrous plant also had the power to *'properly healeth exulterated genitalls'*. This property was first proved in 1996 in a randomised, controlled clinical trial carried out by Dr Tanweer Syed, who studied the effect of topical aloe on the lesions genital of herpes and found that they healed almost 30% faster when treated with aloe, compared with the conventional treatment.

The Aloe Vera plant is readily adaptable and, because man carried it with him from place to place, it made its first recorded appearance in London in 1693. By the early 19th century, and according to chroniclers of the times, many of those that had the wherewithal were enthusiastic users of this so-called "silent healer", and in 1843, 4,227 gourds were imported into the country.

However, despite the fact that physicians had been prescribing it for more than 2,000 years, it wasn't until 1851 that T & H Smith of Edinburgh discovered Aloin. The two Smith brothers believed that small doses of this substance acted as a digestive tonic and had a beneficial influence on the liver; larger doses however, were found to have a marked and even unfortunate laxative effect.

Throughout the 18th and 19th centuries aloe remained one of the most popular of prescribed and over-the-counter medicines.

Aloin is a substance found only in the sap of the Aloe Vera plant. When a leaf is freshly cut, thick yellow orange sap drips out and in ancient times was collected and concentrated. Apart from being used as a powerful laxative, it was also consumed to kill parasites such as worms in the gut so, not only did it relieve constipation, the outcome could be examined to ensure that it had done its job! Later on, this extremely bitter substance was employed by my grandmother, not to rid me of worms, but painted onto my fingers to stop me biting my nails; it tasted so disgusting, it did the job! Another more interesting use for it was by the women of ancient Egypt who painted it on their nipples when they wanted to wean their babies. One mouthful of this dreadful stuff and the baby would be on solids the following day!

These women also thought that the sap of Aloe Vera, containing the aloin, would bring about a miscarriage of an unwanted pregnancy. This was not the case, as modern research on pregnant rats, which behave very similarly to human beings, has shown; despite huge amounts of sap added to their food, they did not miscarry. Unfortunately, some people today still believe this myth and consequently pregnant women are often advised not to take Aloe Vera. Many products do not contain any aloin at all, consequently the presence or absence of Aloin in modern Aloe Vera products is a controversial issue. Some companies filter it out, whereas others leave a little in with apparently varying results, which will be explored in the chapter on 'The Plant and its Structure'. However, even with a tiny amount of aloin in the product, it would still be safe for women who are trying to conceive, those who are pregnant and those who are breast feeding.

The fact remains that the fables and myths surrounding Aloe Vera's history are fascinating, both from a scientific and anecdotal point of view.

For example, the two most famous Egyptian queens, Cleopatra and Nefertiti, were apparently advocates of aloe as part of their extensive beauty regimes. Unfortunately, rather like the mythical baths of asses' milk, this is not genuinely documented and may just be wishful thinking.

Alexander the Great also gets a mention in the aloe hall of fame. Following his conquest of Persia in 333BC, the boy king was said to have been persuaded by his mentor, Aristotle, to capture the island of Socotra in the Indian Ocean. A battle was subsequently fought in an effort to secure the island's famed aloe supplies, so necessary in the treatment of Alexander's wounded troops. I took this tale with a pinch of salt at first, particularly as Alexander is known to have travelled home by land. However, I subsequently learnt that he sent one of his generals home by sea with about 500 soldiers, so maybe Alexander was the victor of Socotra after all.

Explorers Marco Polo and Christopher Columbus also documented the use of Aloe Vera as an important medicine on their voyages.

Another popular myth is that Aloe Vera is referred to in the Bible. In fact it is lignin aloe that is mentioned five times, but not Aloe Vera. The most famous passage comes from St John's Gospel:

'And there came also, Nicodemus, which at the first came to Jesus by night, and brought a mixture of myrrh, and aloes, about a hundred pounds weight...'

Lignin aloe is a tree with a scented bark which was used to make incense, as well as being a main ingredient in ointments the preservation and embalming of the dead.

The true aloe has been endowed with such marvellous properties that, over thousands of years and in many different parts of the world, it has been given almost as many evocative names. I know of no herb with as many similar nicknames from so many different cultures around the world. This must say something. Here are just a selection:

Heaven's Blessing	Plant of Life	Burn Plant
Dietary Plant	Healing Plant	Medicine Plant
Potted Physician	Wonder Plant	Wand of Heaven
First Aid Plant	Silent Healer	Single Bible

The Japanese have a name which caps them all 'ISHA IRAZU' which translated means 'No need for a doctor'.

The Plant and Its Structure

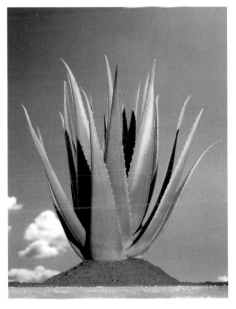

Aloe Vera is often mistaken for a cactus, but is in fact a succulent and one of the spikier members of the lily family. A small bushy plant bearing green, fleshy, tapered leaves, its family is a large one, including about 3,700 species of flowering plants, as well as garlic, onion and asparagus. Aloe Vera itself forms part of a subspecies (the Aloinae) of which there are over 200 types.

Whilst most species are non-toxic, there are about 15 poisonous ones, including one containing a lethal deadly hemlock-like substance, similar to that chosen by Socrates to end his life.

The potency of Aloe Vera is due to its rich variety of ingredients, which are present in perfect balance, and work together as a team. Although the solid portion of the plant forms only 1%-1.5%, the rest being water, this small amount of active ingredient can produce a substantial effect. The only way to account for this is to accept the philosophy of synergism within the plant. Synergism means that the effect of the whole is greater than the effects of the component parts, so although individual members of the team could only have an effect, together they can achieve a great deal more.

There are thought to be only five varieties of the aloe family which possess documented medicinal benefits, and of these it is Aloe Barbadensis Miller,

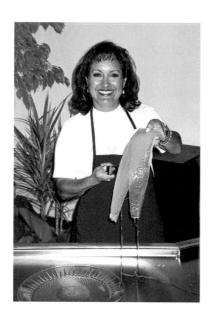

called Aloe Linné, Aloe Vulgaris or the Curacao Aloe, which has been of most use to mankind because it has been shown to be the most powerful of all aloes. The others are:

- Aloe Perryi Baker, the Socotrine Aloe or Zanzibar Aloe;
- Aloe Ferox, often called Cape Aloe;
- Aloe Arborescens
- Aloe Saponaria

The last two, and least popular, are mainly used in Japan.

Aloe Barbadensis Miller is the only species that should be called by the name Aloe Vera (which translates as 'True Aloe'). It was first referred to by this name in a South African publication called Flora Indira by N L Burman in 1768, and in Miller's herbal dictionary later the same year.

The species, which flourishes in warm dry climates, is indigenous to and originated in Africa. However, Aloe Vera plants have travelled widely and are now cultivated both in the near and Far East as well as in the West Indies, where they arrived on the Caribbean island of Barbados in about 1650. They also flourish in the drier parts of Europe, such as Spain.

Aloe Vera's greatest enemy is frost, which rules out any serious cultivation in Northern Europe. However, it should still grow well – if more slowly - in a pot at home. So, when you next get bitten, burnt or stung, simply cut off a leaf, squeeze the gel out from the leaf onto the wound and rub it in. You will soon feel the First Aid Plant work its magic.

Nowadays, although medicines and drugs can be very effective in treating ailments, long- term use can often involve unpleasant side effects. Consequently, increasing numbers of consumers, as well as scientists, are considering more traditional and often more natural therapies which have been neglected for many years. Aloe Vera is just one of those natural solutions and one which is increasingly being highlighted in the media.

The Structure

Aloe Vera takes four to five years to reach maturity, by which time its leaves are about 60cm or two feet in length and about 8-10cm or 3-4 inches wide at the base. The leaves taper to a point and possess soft marginal spines. If the stem is cut transversely, the leaves can be seen growing in a rosette pattern.

From the centre of the mass of dark green leaves, the flower stem develops, reaching about 90cms (three feet) in length, followed by a growth of long, rather tubular yellow flowers in the case of Barbadensis Miller. At the base of the mother plant little suckers, or 'pups', grow and are easily separated to make new cuttings. The plant can of course also reproduce by cross-fertilisation. In the wild, pollination is often performed by humming birds. Hence this successful plant can reproduce both sexually and asexually.

Aloe Vera, being a perennial, has a life span of about 12 years, although the leaves are usually harvested at about three to four years of age. When the outer leaves are harvested, possibly up to three times a year, the plant is able to 'seal' itself against water loss, a protective facility peculiar to succulents. Within a few seconds of being severed, the cut films over and, during the next few minutes, a rubber-like protective coating prevents further loss of sap, stopping the stem from becoming dessicated and enabling the plant to continue living. In a short time, the wound heals completely. Small wonder it has been called The Medicine Plant. Maybe primitive man witnessed this self-healing property and thought "perhaps there is something in this plant that could help heal me."

Inside the Leaf

The structure of the aloe leaf (seen below in cross-section) shows the outer rind.

CROSS SECTION OF THE ALOE VERA LEAF

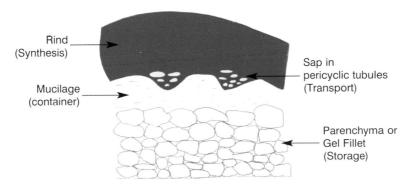

Rind (Synthesis)

Mucilage (container)

Sap in pericyclic tubules (Transport)

Parenchyma or Gel Fillet (Storage)

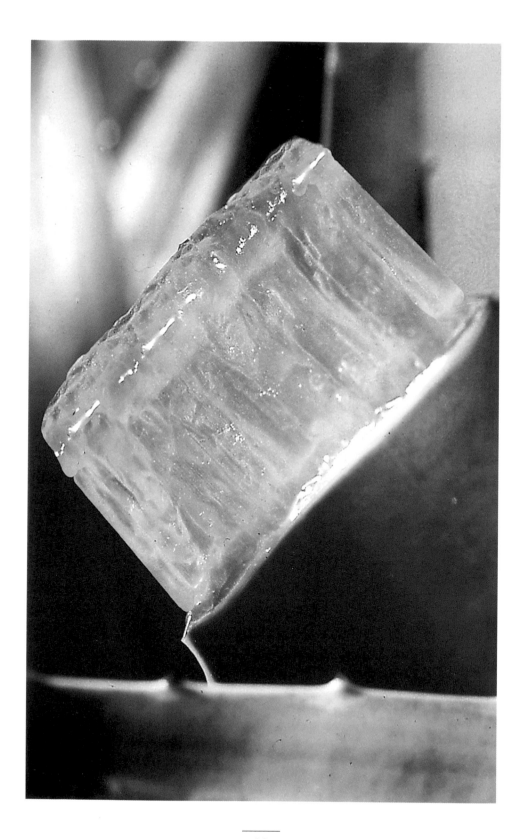

This is about 15 cell layers thick, of a dark green colour, with a hard, waxy surface. The hardness is due to the large amounts of calcium and magnesium present. The colour denotes the presence of chlorophyll which utilises sunlight, carbon dioxide and water in order to manufacture the aloe vera gel. Below the rind are vascular bundles, or tubes, of xylem and phloem. This is the sap, or transport system of the plant, which takes up water and minerals from the roots and transports the products of photosynthesis to be stored in the gel.

When a leaf is cut and held up, sap will quickly drain out of the larger tubules.

The Leaf and its Contents

There are over 75 known ingredients in the Aloe Vera leaf, which are divided into eight distinct categories. I suspect that there are still others to be discovered. However, although there has been some confusion over the exact content of some of the fractions, general consensus, taken from a review of recent literature, is that the solid fraction only forms some 0.5-1.5% of the plant, which is a relatively small amount. Its average pH value is 4.55, which makes it rather acid. In the next chapter, we will explore how and where these ingredients work.

Aloe vera gel is one of nature's most potent cocktails, but in analysing the contents of the Aloe Vera leaf, I shall look at the four basic structures:

1. Rind
2. Sap
3. Mucilage
4. Inner gel

Lignin is a cellulose-based substance found in the gel with no known specific medicinal properties, although its presence in topical aloe preparations are thought to provide the ability to penetrate the human skin.

Saponins are glycosides which are thought to comprise about three per cent of aloe vera gel. They are soapy substances, containing antiseptic properties, which are capable of cleansing.

Minerals

- *Calcium* has an important structural role in bones and teeth, but is also essential for cellular structure and nerve transmission. It requires a balance of phosphorus and magnesium to work effectively, and needs Vitamin D for its absorption.

- *Manganese* is a component of many enzymes and is necessary for the activation of others. These substances are complex proteins, which act as biochemical catalysts, thereby speeding up the route of clinical reaction in the plant.

- *Sodium* is a very important mineral, responsible for preventing body fluids from becoming too acid or too alkaline. It is also involved in the electrical conductivity in muscles and nerves, as well as facilitating the uptake of nutrients by individual cells.

- *Potassium*, like sodium, is involved in the acid-base balance in the body as well as electrical conductivity in nerves and muscles.

- *Copper* is also a component of a number of enzymes and facilitates the action of iron as an oxygen carrier in red blood cells.

- *Magnesium* is intimately involved in the metabolism of calcium during bone formation and is also needed by nerve and muscle membranes to enable them to conduct electrical impulses.

- *Zinc* is involved in major metabolic pathways contributing to the metabolism of proteins, carbohydrates (sugars) and fats. An inadequate intake would have an adverse effect on any tissue which dies and is then renewed rapidly, such as skin, gut lining, or the immune system. Recent studies have shown that schizophrenia may, in part, be associated with zinc deficiency. Zinc is also recognised as a very important factor in men's health and reproductive function.

- *Chromium* is necessary for the proper function of insulin, which in turn controls blood sugar levels. It is therefore vital for diabetics to have sufficient.

- *Iron* is the "haem" part of haemoglobin in red blood cells. It enables oxygen to be transported around the body as oxyhaemoglobin. Iron deficiency anaemia is very common in those with poor nutrition and in any situation where there is depletion through chronic blood loss, e.g. excessive menstruation.

Vitamins

Vitamins A, C & E are the important antioxidant vitamins, essential in the fight against damaging free radicals. All three positively influence the immune system, and Vitamin C in particular assists in wound healing; it also makes collagen, keeping bones skin and joints firm and strong. Vitamin A is essential to maintain normal night vision. Vitamin E helps the body utilise oxygen, prevents blood clots, thrombosis, atherosclerosis. It also improves wound healing and fertility and is good for the skin.

Free radicals are constantly being formed by normal body processes, but they are also produced by any form of combustion such as smoking, exhaust fumes, radiation, and even the burning of food, such as on a barbecue or by frying. They will endeavour to oxidise tissues and can cause a great deal of damage, triggering everything from cancers to cataracts, arterial disease and premature aging. You only have to look at rusty metal to understand the effect that oxygen and oxidisation have.

These oxidising free radicals can be neutralised by Vitamins A, C & E, as well as by the mineral selenium and micro-nutrients called bioflavinoids. There is no doubt that you need to include antioxidants in your diet, and the best natural source has to be fresh fruit and vegetables, especially leafy vegetables such as cabbage and kale, seed bearing vegetables such as broccoli and all varieties of beans.

The B Vitamins, including Choline

These are associated with the production of energy and with amino acid metabolism, which helps develop muscle mass.

Vitamin B12. Aloe Vera is one of the rare plant sources of this essential vitamin necessary for manufacturing red blood cells. A deficiency of Vitamin B12 will eventually lead to anaemia.

Folic Acid. This is very important in the development of blood cells. A deficiency will also cause anaemia.

Amino Acids

The human body requires 20 amino acids for good health to be maintained and all but eight can be manufactured in the body. The others, called essential amino acids, need to be taken as food. Together, they form the building blocks of proteins from which we manufacture and repair muscle.

Aloe Vera provides 19 of the 20 required amino acids and seven of the eight essential ones. The missing amino acid is tryptophan, although Bill Coates, an American pharmacist and Aloe expert, claims it has this one too. The evidence is not conclusive enough for me to agree, although providing seven out of the eight required is good going.

Enzymes

Aloe Vera contains many enzymes (listed below), which can be divided into two groups, those that aid digestion and those that are anti-inflammatory. Of the ones that aid digestion some, like amylase, break down starch and sugar, whilst others, like lipase, help break down fats. Consequently, the nutrients in our food can be more efficiently absorbed, when one is drinking aloe on a regular basis.

Peroxidase	Cellulase	Aliiase
Carboxypeptidase	Catalase	Amylase
Lipase	Alkaline Phosphatase	

Sugars

Aloe Vera contains two sorts of sugars, monosaccharides, such as glucose and fructose, and long chain sugars called polysaccharides, the main one being a glucomannose often referred to as Acemannan.

Sterols

The plant sterols are important anti-inflammatory agents, the three main ones being:

Campesterol	β Sitosterol	Lupeol

Lupeol also acts as an antiseptic and analgesic agent.

Salicylic acid, also found in Aloe Vera, is metabolized in the body to an aspirin-like compound which, together with lupeol, provide some of its pain-killing properties.

Other small molecules found in the solid matter are various plant hormones.

How Does It Work?

Are the positive effects of Aloe Vera just myths or is there medicine at work? Folklore and anecdotal evidence show us what type of conditions it's supposed to help, and research has tried to relate these to general biochemical and physiological principles. To understand this relationship, it's necessary to look at the plant's constituents as well as its chemistry.

We know that the Aloe Vera leaf is approximately 99 per cent water. This means that the total amount of nutrient which remains is only one per cent of the plant. However, this one per cent contains over 75 ingredients which together form a cocktail of all the substances previously mentioned. In their relatively small amounts you might not expect them to have much of an effect, certainly not the many positive results which have been witnessed and recorded. Why is that?

I believe that the answer lies in their synergistic action. Synergism is the combined effect of drugs, organs, and so on, that exceeds the sum of their individual effects. It is this balance that has taken thousands of years to evolve in this extraordinary plant and one which produces its dramatic results; all the constituents work as a team and, together, are able to achieve more.

To produce aloe vera gel, the mature leaves are harvested when the plant is about four years old. The product is either produced from the whole leaf, which is ground up and then filtered to remove the solid matter, eventually passing through carbon filters to extract all the anthraquinone fraction, or the parenchymal plant tissue and mucilage is filleted out of the leaf to produce a gel containing only a minute quantity of sap.

The product is then preserved by subjecting it either to heat or to chemical sterilisation. Various antioxidants such as ascorbic acid are often added. These inhibit the plant enzymes, protecting the tissue, and particularly its phenolic components, from being oxidized, which would darken the product. Other ingredients, such as preservatives, along with thickening and flavouring agents - preferably naturally sourced – are added. All these ingredients help stabilise the end product by retarding microbial contamination, as well as chemical and physical changes.

The stabilised gel is then made up into health drinks, or topical cremes and lotions, where it exerts its influence in two main areas: membranes and surfaces, known anatomically as epithelial tissue, such as the skin, or on the immune system.

I believe that the best quality products result from a filleting process rather than a wholeleaf process and where the stabilisation process is a 'cold' one where excessive damaging heat is not used.

ITS USES

In my experience as a family doctor, I have found aloe vera gel to be particularly effective when used on burns, where it soothes, relieves pain, reduces inflammation and promotes healing, with minimal scar formation.

I have also seen several of my patients with conditions such as chronic leg ulcers, chronic itching, eczema, psoriasis and acne benefit from the treatment, which can sometimes be used as a safe alternative to steroid cremes. This is important because the prolonged use of more powerful steroids has several undesirable side effects.

Aloe Vera is also extremely useful to the cosmetics industry, partly because of its ability to penetrate tissue due to its lignin content, and partly due to its anaesthetic, antibacterial, antiviral, antifungal and anti-inflammatory effects.

Aloe Vera's effect on the skin is therefore as a healing and anti-aging agent, because of its ability to moisturise, reduce wrinkling through increased formation of collagen and elastin, and to reduce pigment formation. It can also be formulated as a sunscreen, when it not only blocks ultraviolet light, but also enhances the skin's immune reaction to these damaging rays.

Other traditional uses for Aloe Vera, as if all the above weren't enough, include conditions involving damaged tissue found in asthma, where the lining of the bronchioles becomes inflamed and swollen, as well as stomach and bowel problems. Irritable bowel syndrome, for example, responds particularly well to aloe vera gel.

ALOE VERA HAS THREE IMPORTANT QUALITIES:

It provides essential micro nutrients

Tissues that die and are rapidly renewed, such as the lining of the gut which renews itself approximately every four days, and skin which renews itself every 21 to 28 days or so, need a rich and ready supply of building materials to produce and maintain healthy and efficient cells. A poor diet, and one which is deficient in certain key elements, will not produce a fit and healthy body or mind.

It has become apparent that the tendency of many people today, particularly children, to eat junk food, is causing deficiency states which can only contribute towards a generation of unhealthy adults. Increasing numbers of doctors are emphasising that good nutrition is the basis of good health and that many diseases can be treated quickly and effectively by changes in diet, rather than with drugs, which often treat only the symptoms and not the underlying cause.

With the increasing importance of nutritional medicine it is often said that 'if the doctors of today don't become the nutritionists of tomorrow then the nutritionists of today will become the doctors of tomorrow'.

It kills bacteria, viruses, fungi and yeasts

Experiments in the laboratory have been carried out on numerous organisms and have regularly shown that, at normal strength, aloe vera gel can either destroy (bactericidal) or inhibit the growth (bacteriostatic) of several bacterial organisms, especially those that cause skin and wound infections, such as the dreaded Staphylococcus.

The first real investigation of the anti-microbial action of Aloe Vera took place in the USA between 1968 and 1972, when two doctors, Zimmerman and Sims, studied the effect of stabilised gel on Staphylococcus, as well as other organisms including the yeast Candida, the cause of many problems, especially in women. They discovered that Aloe Vera inhibited growth of the bacteria in 70% concentration and candida (yeast) at a 50% concentration.

In 1970, they tested it against the fungi which causes Athlete's Foot (tinea pedis). Two of these particularly unattractive fungi that can affect both toe and finger-nails, were both destroyed in an 85% solution of Aloe Vera. Further testing

---

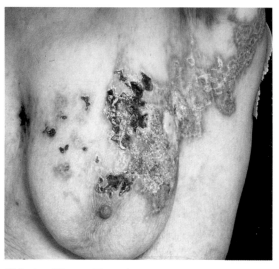
Shingles (Herpes Zoster).

showed it to be virucidal to Herpes Simplex, as well as to the painful and persistent Herpes Zoster (shingles).

Further excitement was to come. In 1971, they found that this versatile plant was also shown to destroy Trichomonas Vaginalis, a common cause of sexually transmitted vaginal infection, producing soreness and discharge.

In her summary, Dr Sims reported, 'Aloe Vera is bactericidal to at least six species of bacteria, especially to the more common staphylococcal and streptococcal infections where it is effective in its use on burns patients. In 80 per cent concentration, it is broadly virucidal. It is virucidal to four members of the Herpes strain, including Herpes Simplex and Herpes Zoster. In 80% concentration it is fungicidal against yeast infections, Trichomonas and Candida'.

It is clear from these findings, and others since, that Aloe Vera has the ability to destroy organisms that tend to invade damaged skin and wounds, and which delay and possibly prevent healing.

It reduces inflammation

Inflammation is the response of healthy tissues to injury. The process is a complicated but organised one, involving changes in the local blood supply. The walls of the blood vessels change so that molecules and cells of the immune system may pass through them, thus bringing about clotting, the mounting of an attack on invading organisms and starting of the repair process.

If, however, the inflammatory process is impaired as, for example, in a hypersensitive reaction such as allergic asthma, there will be an adverse effect and further tissue damage will result. If the inflammation is also inappropriate, such as when the body's own tissues are attacked such as in rheumatoid arthritis, for example, the problem will be aggravated. This potentially serious and degenerative condition is generally treated with synthetic drugs to reduce inflammation and thereby pain and stiffness – the non steroidal anti inflammatory drugs. A common NSAID is the over-the-counter Ibuprofen. Whilst these types of drugs are highly effective in reducing symptoms, they can produce nasty side effects, from indigestion, to more extreme conditions such as bleeding stomach ulcers, and even death if the ulcer bursts.

In November, 1995, a report appeared in the British medical press suggesting that about 5% of duodenal, and a massive 22% of gastric ulcers, were associated with the use of non-steroidal anti-inflammatory drugs, yet they continue to be prescribed in their millions. Thousands of people begin with one debilitating condition, are treated, and end up with a second. It is therefore a godsend to find a natural anti-inflammatory agent that works without producing these distressing and potentially fatal side effects.

The positive combination of nutrients, a reduction in infection and inflammation, where appropriate, leads to the promotion of new cell growth and more rapid healing. In a simple laboratory experiment in 1988, aloe vera gel was added to human fibroblast cell culture. There was an eight-fold increase in their replication, over control cultures to which no Aloe Vera had been added.

Fibroblasts are one of the most important types of cells involved in the healing process. They produce the collagen fibres of the scar tissue which knit wounds together, so the more that are working at the site of the injury the better. This may be the single most important factor influenced by Aloe Vera in the acceleration of the healing process.

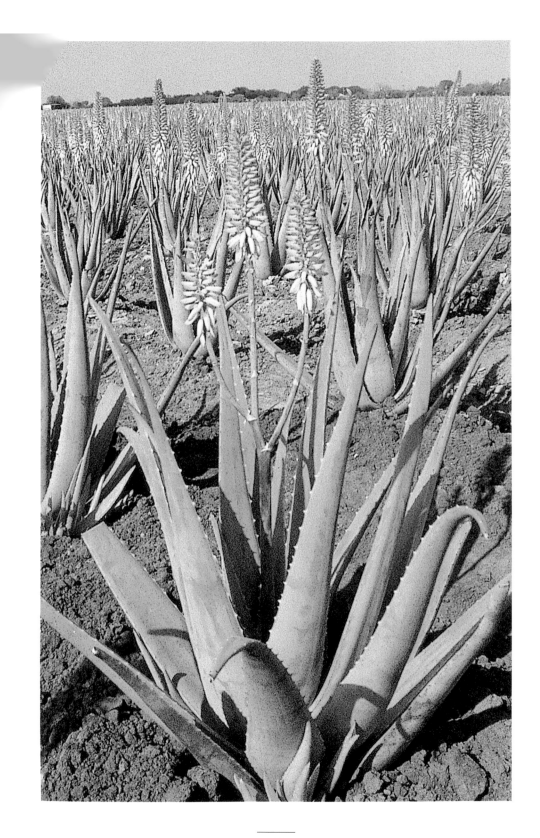

WHAT KIND OF ALOE?

I believe the most fitting description about what type of Aloe to use was supplied by American physician, Dr Ivan Danhof, who said:

"The best aloe is a preparation which maximises the desired constituents, minimises any ingredient with negative effects, maintains the constituents in an unaltered and active form, preserves the actions and benefits, and is present in the final product in amounts which, indeed, can bring about the desired result when the product is used as recommended."

For the present, I think that the best form of aloe is 100% pure stabilised aloe vera gel taken as a health drink. This stabilised gel should also be the major ingredient of any topical product such as shampoos, cremes and ointments, lotions and sprays.

Aloe Vera is currently grown commercially, mainly in the Rio Grande Valley in Texas, USA, in the Philippines, the Dominican Republic, South Africa, Spain and in Australia. There are several aloe companies marketing a variety of aloe compounds, some excellent and some which I believe are quite useless. For any Aloe Vera drink to stand a chance of doing good, it needs to contain a substantial quantity of the parenchymatous gel. If a product is clear, looks like water and tastes like water, then it probably is water, and not particularly beneficial.

There is an independent organization established in the USA called International Aloe Science Council which, amongst other things, evaluates the quality of aloe products. If such products meet with various criteria and reach a particular standard, they are accredited with the IASC seal of approval, as shown. This mark of quality can then appear on the container. I suggest that any aloe products which do not display this seal of approval may not do much good.

Cold stabilized aloe vera gel, which is my preferred preparation, is about 97% pure and the nearest thing that you can get to the natural raw gel extracted from the plant. As I have said, it is extremely safe and non-toxic, although when people first start to take the gel it may stir them up in more ways than one. Some people may experience a change in bowel habit for a few days, together

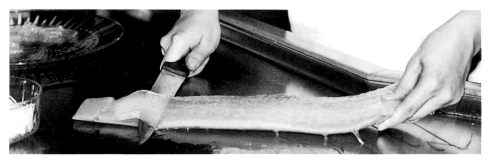
Hand filleting of aloe.

with mild abdominal discomfort, but this should soon pass. Some people refer to this initial phase as one of detoxification, but I think this is a misnomer because it is merely the effect of aloe of the gut.

Currently, the main debate continues about the relative benefits of aloe vera gel versus whole leaf aloe but, like many others, I think it important to find the nearest we can to the raw gel.

In the production of whole leaf aloe products, the entire plant is harvested and crushed, rather than just the individual leaves. Solid matter, including the pulverised rind, is separated and the resultant fluid is passed through carbon filters to remove the anthraquinones. It is often then concentrated for a less weighty product, thus reducing transportation costs thereby reducing the retail price as well as retail costs. This is often stated to be a better product because it contains more polysaccharides than the natural gel. However, I believe this argument is flawed. The reason is that there are only a limited number of specialised cells lining the small bowel capable of absorbing this long chain sugar whole, without the need for it to be broken down by enzymatic action, so any extra polysaccharide in the product over and above the capacity of these cells to absorb it is therefore wasted. I believe there only need to be about 1200-1400 mg/lt in a product to get maximum absorption.

Quite apart from this, it's possible that when the fluid is passed through the fine carbon filters during the manufacturing process, unknown, unidentified and possibly important elements are also filtered out.

So far, there is no real evidence to support whole leaf aloe being superior to 100% stabilised aloe vera gel, and I'm inclined to support this. I believe that many of the considerations that go into the making of whole leaf aloe are commercial ones which aim to produce a cheaper product for a greater profit margin. So, the choice is yours.

Where Does It Work?

Aloe Vera is not a cure-all, it merely suppresses symptoms and, despite claims over the centuries of the miraculous medical powers it possesses, it has actually been found to work on just two main areas. The first includes surfaces and membranes, such as the skin and the lining of the sinuses, nose, throat, stomach and bowel, together with the linings of the lungs and genital tract. Secondly, it works on the immune system, which is designed to protect the body from attack by external aggressors such as bacteria, viruses and fungi, as well as internal threats from other enemies such as cancer cells.

SURFACES AND MEMBRANES

The skin is a vital body organ protecting everything contained within it. It allows us to sense heat and cold, touch and pain and, through variations in blood supply and sweating, helps control our body temperature and fluid loss. The largest organ in the body, it accounts for 16% of the body's total weight and, despite exposure to all manner of adverse conditions and ill treatment, from inside and out, it is remarkably resilient. However, prolonged exposure to the extremes of weather and external pollution, poor nutrition, and the effects of internal stress, can result in damage and premature aging and the tendency to develop disorders such as eczema, psoriasis and, more seriously, ulcers and even skin cancer.

Aloe vera gel has proved helpful in treating a number of these more serious conditions, as well as more every day problems such as insect bites, stings, bruises, blisters and burns.

It is refreshing that doctors are increasingly using Aloe Vera to treat certain conditions in their practices. However, although the sceptics amongst them may not use it themselves, they are now more likely to let their patients buy it.

The anatomical word for surfaces and membranes is 'epithelium'. For damaged epithelium to receive the benefits of Aloe Vera, the gel can be taken orally. It can also be applied topically to the damaged skin experienced with eczema or psoriasis. However, general dermatological principles must still be followed. If the skin is dry, it needs to be moisturised, and therefore any product should have an emollient or greasy base. If the skin is oily, a non-greasy or drying base needs to be used. Water and alcohol-based lotions are best used in hairy areas and dressings are generally needed where the skin is ulcerated.

On a personal note, to illustrate Aloe Vera's effect on chronically inflamed membranes, I discovered to my absolute joy that, after taking it daily for about two weeks, my nasal catarrh - the legacy of smoking 20 cigarettes a day for 23 years – was much reduced and because my breathing was made easier, my wife announced that I was no longer snoring as much; so Aloe Vera can even improve marital harmony!

Delighted as I am with both results, I am aware that if I stop using Aloe Vera, the problem recurs after a week or so, as it only suppresses the symptoms and is not a permanent cure for the problem.

My wife has also benefitted. Being an enthusiastic cook, she is always burning her hands and arms when she inadvertently catches them on the hot doors of our Aga oven, but a swift application of Aloe Vera not only alleviates the pain almost instantly but, with repeated applications, the wounds heal much faster without scarring. Previous burns have left her with multiple small scars on her hands and wrists but at least now she is not adding to them. You can see why Aloe Vera has been called 'The Burn Plant'. My wife is now so confident that she is even less concerned about wearing the protective gloves provided by Aga, for she knows that if she does burn herself she can get some very quick and efficient relief!!

With experience, my usage of Aloe Vera in my general medical practice has slowly increased in recent years, especially in areas where my usual treatment has failed or not been particularly successful, where there have been side effects, or where the patient has been keen to use 'something natural'.

In my experience, skin conditions which respond most positively are:

Acne vulgaris and rosacea

Eczema, especially atopic eczema in young children

Seborrhoeic dermatitis

Psoriasis

Chronic urticaria

Ulcers

Athlete's Foot

I made an important observation when I conducted an experiment in treating a large ulcer on the shin of an elderly lady, with nothing but topical Aloe Vera. The shin is a notoriously difficult place for an ulcer because it can take a long time to heal, whatever treatment is used. In this instance, the ulcer was the result of a trauma from knocking her leg against a sharp corner on a piece of furniture. I was lucky enough to treat it within a few hours of the accident happening and, after cleansing the wound, persuaded my nursing staff to apply Aloe Vera twice a day beneath a moist dressing.

The speed of the healing was quite remarkable, with no sign of infection, often a dreaded complication. My nurses were also impressed and, as a result, planned to use it again on some of their more difficult cases. Quite remarkably, this particular ulcer healed with minimal scarring, a typical feature of aloe treatment.

If a result such as this is indeed consistent, then the Aloe Vera approach could save the National Health Service a considerable amount of money. Other health workers have also reported excellent results with similar treatment of burns and ulcers, and in the USA it is used regularly in many major burns units.

Cosmetic skin preparations are increasingly sold 'with Aloe Vera' as the handle, when they are designed to nourish the skin and retard the effects of aging. Both Roots the chemists and the Body Shop have used it for some years and, more recently, Gillette has added Aloe Vera to one of its products, ostensibly to make shaving a more pleasant experience for men – and some women. The combination of high quality aloe in preparations firstly helps to moisturise and soften the skin and, by penetration, promotes an anti-inflammatory and anti-aging effect. The latter includes a reduction and sometimes eradication of 'liver spots' on older skin.

Secondly, after penetration, it stimulates cells called fibroblasts in the dermis to produce more collagen and elastin fibres, thereby reducing wrinkling, which occurs as a result of reduced collagen levels. Finally, it enhances the skin's immune system, therefore lessening the risk of damage from ultra-violet rays.

It must be said that even Aloe Vera can have some side effects, although these are more likely to be of the welcome variety. Women in particular, after several weeks of using the gel, often remark that their nails grow more quickly and are less brittle, that their hair also grows faster and looks healthier, and that because Aloe Vera has a vasodilatory effect (expanding the blood vessels in the skin), they can develop rosy cheeks. When people are told they look well, they often feel well as a result.

THE LINING OF THE DIGESTIVE TRACT

The other major body system which has been consistently helped by Aloe Vera is the digestive tract, where it has successfully treated conditions ranging from simple indigestion and heartburn, to peptic and duodenal ulcers, the potentially more serious diverticulitis, ulcerative colitis, and Crohn's Disease.

As I've already said, the sap of Aloe Vera was used widely as a purgative and a general aid to digestion, but it is the anti-inflammatory and wound-healing effects found in the gel that benefited the sufferers of inflammatory bowel conditions such as colitis and diverticulitis. Many have reported positive results with regular use of Aloe Vera. However, as with skin problems, their symptoms tend to return after stopping the treatment, so taking aloe vera gel needs to be part of an ongoing regime. These conditions are well known for relapsing and remitting, and for those who have suffered regularly from these unpleasant complaints, the reduced frequency and severity of the relapses has been benefit enough. I am often asked if Aloe Vera is available as a suppository but, as far as I'm aware, it's not as yet. Maybe it's in the pipeline!

Irritable Bowel Syndrome is a condition which I think deserves a special mention. It is now the most common disorder of the bowel in the industrialised western world and the most frequent cause for referral to a gastroenterologist by GPs. It is estimated that there may be more than five million sufferers in the UK alone.

IBS presents as a number of symptoms that vary from person to person, with the most common features being abdominal pain and bloating, diarrhoea and/or constipation. There is seldom an effect on the person's general health and the sufferers usually maintain their weight. However, it can be an extremely debilitating and embarrassing condition, and can also prevent sufferers from going out, getting on with their work, or even their lives. It is often associated with stress and anxiety, emotional upset and depression, and may be found in combination with other 'irritable' organs, such as the bladder.

Conventional treatment is not very effective and depends on dietary change, usually with an increase in fibre, anti-diarrhoea or bulking agents, anti-spasmodic drugs, anti-depressants, and counselling and/or hypnotherapy. Many of these measures are tried, sometimes in combination, because the condition is not yet fully understood. Some think the condition is due to a disorder of the bowel's regular and smooth peristaltic movements – a 'dysmotility', and others claim that the gut's sensitivity is decreased. Another theory is that there is too much yeast, such as Candida Albicans, in the bowel, which may be the underlying cause. Yet another group of doctors, as with post-viral fatigue syndrome [M.E.], think it's a psychosomatic response to the stresses of modern living. I'm sure there is no doubt that such stressors do exacerbate IBS, but it is hard to know precisely how much of a role they do play.

The latest research tends to suggest that with many sufferers it is the aftermath of having taken inappropriately prescribed or bought antibiotics for conditions such as Travellers' Diarrhoea. This condition should really just be treated with rest and fluids and will generally settle in a day or two when the gut flora settles down.

Whatever the cause, in 1995 the British Medical Journal rather dishearteningly stated: 'No uniformly successful treatment exists for the Irritable Bowel Syndrome'.

I know from experience that there are a lot of dissatisfied patients out there. When the journalist Hazel Courtney wrote an article on IBS in the Daily Mail in 1994 featuring, amongst others, my views on Aloe Vera, it generated thousands of letters from sufferers asking for more information.

Today, Aloe Vera is my first-line approach in the treatment of confirmed IBS and I have more success with this regime than with any other. Unfortunately, it is not successful in every case and I suspect that failures tend to occur more when the emotional response to stress is greatest, i.e. there is less of a physical component. But it is greatly reassuring and pleasing to hear patients say, as one did, 'I can now go shopping with confidence – it's great!' Previously she could only shop where she

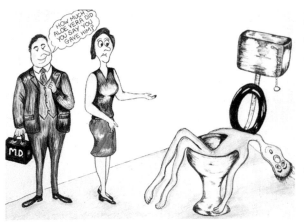

knew there was an abundance of strategically placed toilets.

I must emphasise that I am talking about aloe vera gel, not the old 'bitter aloes' made from the sap. This would produce quite different and potentially disastrous results!

IMMUNE SYSTEM

Those who take aloe vera gel regularly, including myself, report a greater sense of well being. They seem to feel generally better and more at ease. I believe this comes about because of a well-balanced and effective immune system, so fewer coughs, colds and sore throats.

As the immune system exists to protect the body from change caused by invading organisms, for example, bacteria, viruses or altered cells such as cancer cells, its efficient functioning is vital. It is a complex system, involving many different elements which I do not claim to fully understand, since the study of immunology is a subject in its own right. So I will present it in a greatly over-simplified form in which I shall mention only the key players. There is a whole lot more going on in the background which modifies the action of these key cells; they do not work in isolation.

The immune system works around the clock to protect the body from attack. Therefore any disruption to its immediate and efficient response is likely to cause a major problem to the individual. Problems can arise where the immune system is underactive, or even when there is inappropriate action such as when the system attacks the host tissues. Such an action will cause so-called auto immune disorders such as ulcerative colitis, rheumatoid arthritis and lupus.

If the immune system is unable to produce an adequate response, the individual can't fight infection and will eventually succumb to illness or disease. The classic instance of such a situation is, of course, AIDS or Acquired Immune Deficiency Syndrome. This is harmful enough to ultimately cause death, as it can when the body reacts overwhelmingly to certain food allergies, such as we see in the increasing problem of peanut allergy in children, when they develop anaphylactic shock. This reaction is the worst possible form of hypersensitivity, where the sufferer collapses within seconds of eating the particular food and is in grave danger of dying unless adrenalin is immediately to hand. Most people who are known to have a tendency to this severe form of allergy carry around with them self-injectable forms of adrenalin, since there is no time to wait for the doctor or the ambulance. Therefore it is vital that the response should be just enough to knock out the enemy without going over the top.

Such immune responses continuously occur in healthy individuals. The immune system should be thought of as an essential part of our defence mechanism, continually repelling and destroying invaders and abnormal cells as they appear.

The Key Players

The most important cells are called lymphocytes, of which there are two main types, B cells and T cells, found in lymphoid tissue and in the blood.

Almost as important are cells called phagocytes, which are basically scavengers. Some of these are found in tissue, whilst others which are the white blood cells, are found circulating in the blood. B lymphocytes produce antibodies, but the T lymphocytes have several functions in that they seem to orchestrate the response of the system.:

- They help the cells to make antibodies
- They recognise and destroy cells infected with viruses
- They activate phagocytes or scavenger cells to take up pathogens that they have identified
- They control the level and quality of the immune system

As you can see, life appears to be a constant fight, both internally and externally. I see the immune response as a battle in which orders are delivered by chemical messengers, called cytokines. The cytokine systems orchestrate the T helper cells (lymphocytes) to search out and destroy the enemy. It is at this level where the polysaccharide Acemannan, a major component of Aloe Vera found in the mucilage layer, works.

This important component, Acemannan, is found amongst the sugar fraction of the plant. It is a long chain polysaccharide and acts as an immunomodulator, which means it has the ability to either enhance or to slow down the immune response. This remarkable activity has been demonstrated and is well

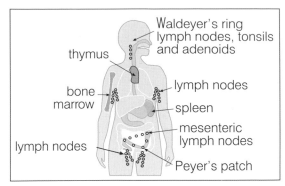

Diagram labels:
- thymus
- Waldeyer's ring lymph nodes, tonsils and adenoids
- bone marrow
- lymph nodes
- spleen
- mesenteric lymph nodes
- lymph nodes
- Peyer's patch

documented in laboratory experiments.

I have suggested its use for my patients with post viral fatigue syndrome on an empirical basis, and several have benefitted. Whilst the numbers so far are too small for me to be able to draw any conclusions, since there is no other convincing treatment, it is surely worth a try.

On the basis of what has been said, it would be expected that those suffering from asthma of an allergic origin would benefit from Aloe Vera, either for its immunomodulating or natural anti-inflammatory effect. In general, I have found this to be the case, leading to a reduction in the number of times an inhaler is needed and the reduction in the frequency of severe disabling attacks. As with post viral syndrome, I haven't seen a sufficient number of cases to be absolutely sure about it, but it certainly calls for some research – a topic I'll discuss at the end of the book.

Finally, on this subject, I must tell you Alison's story. Alison is the young woman to whom my first book on this subject was dedicated and the patient who convinced me that there really was something worthwhile in Aloe Vera.

I treated Alison, a delightful young woman, for 15 years. She suffers with Stills disease, or juvenile rheumatoid arthritis. This condition has been progressive since she was a child and, because of its severity and the deformity it has caused, she has been under regular specialist supervision, receiving a variety of potent conventional treatments, both drug treatments, including high-dose non-steroidal anti-inflammatory drugs (NSAIDS) and hydrotherapy. She has borne her disability bravely but several years ago she came to my surgery complaining that, whilst she needed more anti-inflammatories to control her pain and stiffness, she was unable to take any more because of the abdominal pain they caused. a typical Catch 22 situation. I didn't know what else to suggest, so I said: 'You wouldn't like to try a sort of wacky cactus juice that is supposed to have a natural anti-inflammatory effect, as well as settling stomachs, would you?'

Both Alison, and her mother, who was present during the consultation, said they would try anything as long as Alison could get some relief. Unfortunately, I couldn't prescribe it so she had to buy it from a local agent and shortly afterwards, started a course of aloe vera gel.

It was agreed that she would not initially reduce her current level of drugs, but would add the Aloe Vera, and record the amount of NSAIDS she took, and the amount of Aloe Vera, as well as her symptoms, on a daily basis. I was to see her every two weeks.

After a few weeks, we were both thrilled to see an improvement. Her abdominal pain disappeared, she had less joint pain and she certainly looked better and happier, even to the extent of having rosy cheeks for the first time. Over subsequent months she started to reduce her NSAID level until, eighteen months down the road, she was taking about half the amount she used to, still with no side effects. Her quality of life improved considerably and, witnessing the change, albeit in only one patient, but one of the most difficult therapeutically, was the turning point in both my medical career and in my life.

Thank you Alison.

This type of arthritis is, I suspect, helped by a combination of anti-inflammatory and immunomodulatory factors. However, I like many others, have found that Aloe Vera also seems helpful in osteoarthritis, the 'wear and tear' arthritis, which means that the use of aloe in both cases is worth investigating.

We have looked at Acemannan, but there are other positive aspects of polysaccharides, according to American nutritionist, Dr E Harendal. They are found in every single cell in the body and play a crucial role by:

- Lining the colon to prevent absorption of toxic waste
- Providing a life-saving barrier against microbial invasion for each cell, especially viruses
- Providing critical lubrication of joints
- Helping to maintain the capacity of movement of fluids
- Allowing the transfer of gases to the lungs
- Facilitating the absorption of water, electrolytes and nutrients in the gastro intestinal tract

Dr Harendal made the most important statement that his belief is that polysaccharides are as vital to a healthy body as bricks are to a house.

Common Problems Helped By
ALOE VERA

As has been said Aloe Vera works on linings and membranes or epithelial tissue, and the skin is the biggest epithelial organ of the body. From both my own and other people's experiences, often supported by clinical trials or experiments, several conditions have emerged as being helped considerably either by oral ingestion of Aloe Vera drink, by topical application or, as is often the case, by both.

ECZEMA

Eczema can be divided into two types, the type that comes from within

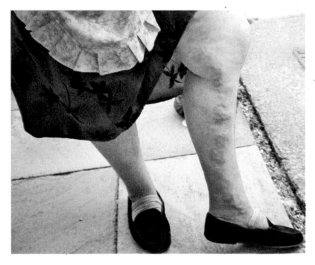

Varicose eczema before Aloe Vera treatment.

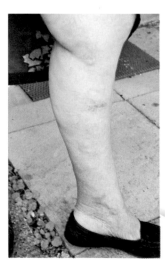

After treatment.

(endogenous), or as a result of external factors, such as allergy, or from irritants (exogenous). Eczema from irritants is usually referred to as dermatitis, but it is the same pathological process. When eczema is present, virtually from birth, it is called juvenile or 'atopic' eczema, and is often linked to asthma and hayfever, which appears in later life.

Eczema is an inflammation of the skin, which can be sudden in onset, i.e. acute with blister formation and weeping ('wet eczema'), or it can be chronic and dry with red thickened patches and very itchy. Scratching leads to more itching, to more scratching, and a vicious circle is built up. Fifty per cent of children with atopic eczema grow out of it, but others go on to develop the chronic form.

The basis of treatment for both the atopic and chronic form:

1. Avoid the use of all soap and use an emollient soap substitute instead.
2. Reduce the dryness of the skin by using moisturiser. This in itself will reduce the itchiness.

3. Use an anti-inflammatory creme.
4. Use a topical antibiotic if there is a possibility of infection, to avoid it spreading as it would.

The anti-inflammatory and anti pruritic (itch) action of Aloe Vera in a moisturising base, such as Lanolin, combined with the natural antibiotic from the beehive, Bee Propolis, is therefore my treatment of choice. Applied three times per day it will often obviate the need for steroid cremes; one of the conventional mainstays of treatment for this difficult condition. Drinking Aloe Vera at the same time will also help provide the newly forming skin cells at the base of the epidermis with the micro-nutrients they need to develop into strong, healthy cells.

The last tip I would give is to add good quality bath oil to the bath water or, in severe cases, coat the body in emulsifying ointment (available over the counter from the pharmacists) before bathing.

Case Study - Eczema

After using aloe propolis creme twice daily for three to four weeks on our nine-year old daughter's eczema, the eczema patches disappeared! However it did get worse before it got better and it was important that we persevered at that point. We understand that this was a 'healing crisis', when the damaged skin cells are pushed up to the surface by the deeper layer of healing skin. We continue to use the creme to keep the condition at bay.

The creme has anti-bacterial, anti-fungal and anti-inflammatory properties, but without the side effects of hydrocortisone cremes. It also moisturises as it heals and is easily absorbed as well, so two jobs are done at once.

The lignins in aloe carry the creme deep into the dermis, promoting healing from that level. Lighter cremes do not penetrate so far and whilst ointment may do, it is far sticker. Aloe has also been found to leave less scarring in the healing process.

A tube of aloe propolis is 2 ½ times the size of a normal tube of prescribed hydrocortisone and is therefore more cost-effective than prescription drugs. As a mother, I am quite happy to pay for my children to have a safe and effective alternative to steroid cremes.

John and Juliet Ross

PSORIASIS

Like Eczema, this condition is more common than people think, because it can appear in many forms. It is in fact a general disorder of the immune system with skin manifestations, anything from a little flakiness of the scalp to large raised red plaques affecting the whole body. The disorder is often familial and can be exacerbated by stress, alcohol consumption and digestive problems.

Whilst various Aloe Vera products, including shampoos, topical cremes and gels, can soothe the rashes, it is the drinking gels that play a key part because of their

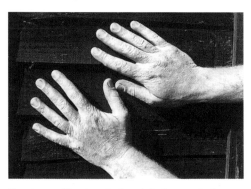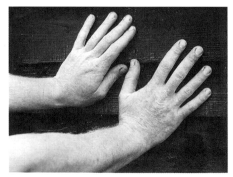

Psoriases affecting the hands before and after treatment.

effect on the immune system. Sometimes the Psoriasis just disappears but, regrettably, not in all cases. Because Psoriasis is a collection of symptoms which vary in different people, it is referred to as a syndrome, and I believe it is only certain types of Psoriasis that can be helped. Any research that could determine which sub-group was most susceptible would be both interesting and important. Those wishing to try the Aloe Vera approach should drink no less than 100mls and as much as 250mls per day. They must do this every day, since Aloe Vera is only a suppressant and the problem will recur if the drink is stopped.

Case Study - Psoriasis

I have suffered from chronic psoriasis for seven years. One morning whilst shaving, I noticed a small circular scale over my right ear. Then, when having a haircut, I noticed more scales around my hairline.

My doctor informed me that it was psoriasis. He explained that it was an ailment for which there was no cure and that very little was known about its actual cause. He recommended coal tar treatments called Oxipor. Rather than heal my condition, it made it worse and I broke out in new areas; eight months later my whole body was covered.

During this time I'd made numerous visits to skin specialists. I was put on various treatments, all cortisone-based, namely Diprosone, Betnovate, Dernovate and others. At this point, my body was raw and bleeding and the itch was almost unbearable.

For six years I never went out in public without wearing a long-sleeved garment and, because my shirt was red with blood, I also had to wear a jacket. The trauma and mental depression I went through were dreadful. At this point, I decided to find out as much about Psoriasis as possible. After a lot of research, I came to the conclusion that the side effects of Cortisone far outweighed the benefits, which in my case were none.

In my view, there are no chemical answers to this problem because the amount of chemical and toxins consumed by us each day are far too high. I always believed that the answer had to come from within because it was from there that the problem began. I tried various herbalists for a cure but once again to no avail.

One evening a friend called to say he might be able to help. He gave me a container of aloe vera gel, some aloe activator, some propolis creme, bath gelee and a loofah. He advised me to take two fluid ounces of gel three times daily, to apply the activator and propolis creme twice daily, and to bath once a day using the bath gelee and loofah to remove the scales.

I began the treatment on the Thursday evening and, to my sheer and utter disbelief, by Friday morning the itch had completely disappeared. I rang Michael straight away with the good news. I applied the activator and propolis creme daily and within five days I could see a vast improvement.

The second week my skin flared up considerably for four days. After this, white patches of new skin began to emerge all over my body and thus I understood that healing had begun. These white patches grew larger and larger until three to four weeks later, my body was virtually clear. Pimples and spots of varying sizes appeared; these are what I called 'secondaries'.

I am now at the stage where I have been taking the gel for six weeks and my body is clearing up at a steady pace. I have no doubt that I have found the answer to my problem and it is my dearest wish that I might be able to help thousands of people who also suffer silently with these problems.

I must also stress that, in my experience, alcohol greatly inhibited the healing process, so I abstained completely. I would strongly advise anyone on this treatment to do likewise until the course of treatment is complete.

I believe in my heart that we owe a great debt of gratitude to those who have given us an array of high quality natural healing products which cause no side effects.

Finbarr Lehane

ACNE

There are two main types, common acne (vulgaris) and acne rosacea. The former affects younger people and is often present in a greasy skin. The skin lesions include blackheads or 'zits', pustules and cysts. There can also often be a lot of residual scarring.

Acne is the result of hormonal change coupled with bacterial action. Rosacea on the other hand, affects older people and presents as a red face with

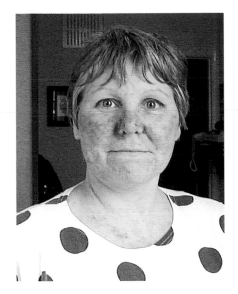 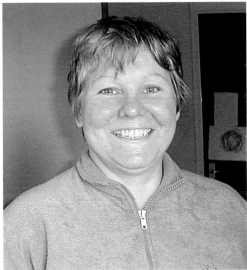

Acne Rosacea before treatment.   After treatment.

occasional pustules. Its cause is not really understood, but it is often made worse by alcohol, spicy food and high emotion.

Both conditions respond to a topical non-greasy Aloe Vera product such as a clear gelly, but with acne vulgaris various lifestyle issues must also be addressed. The skin must be washed regularly and the scalp kept clean. Plenty of sleep, exercise and exposure to UV light are all important, as is drinking enough water – experts recommend around 1 litre a day – to keep the skin hydrated. There must be no squeezing of spots, in order to prevent the spread of infection and scarring.

Case Study - Acne

I am an eighteen-year-old who has suffered with acne for the past three years. It has been so bad that I was prescribed courses of antibiotics throughout the winter. Although this helped to clear up the acne, I wasn't allowed to take the tablets during the summer because of an adverse reaction with sunlight so, by the following winter, the acne was back with a vengeance. That winter, my mother joined a multi level marketing company and started me on bee propolis and garlic thyme tablets, as well as a drink containing aloe vera gel with glucosamine and chondroitin for my long-standing knee injury.

To begin with, I was very sceptical and keen to go back on the antibiotics, but my mother asked me to give the new regime a real chance to work. I can honestly say that over the last two months I have noticed a big difference and now I do not need to be persuaded to continue with the tablets. Also, I am having physiotherapy for my knee injury and the aloe drink seems to be speeding up my recovery.

Andrew McBain

BURNS

One of the aliases given to Aloe Vera is 'The Burn Plant' and with good reason. Serious research into the wound healing qualities of Aloe Vera began as far back as the 1930s. It was found that fresh aloe was able to not only alleviate itching and burning, but that it also helped to regenerate the skin and eliminate scarring.

Subsequently, other experiments followed using both human and animal models, where immediate and delayed histopathological changes of the skin in aloe-treated and non aloe-treated wounds were observed.

The conclusions were that Aloe Vera was able to block the formation of Thromboxane A2, a substance normally found in burnt tissue. Thus, Aloe Vera improved the chance of tissue survival following either burn or frostbite injury by acting as a vaso-dilator, allowing more blood to reach the tissue. As well as the anti-infammatory effect so vital for successful wound healing, aloe was also found to relieve a lot of the pain associated with burns.

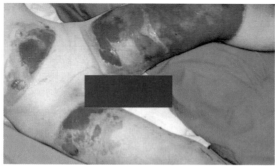

Severe first and second degree burns just after the accident.

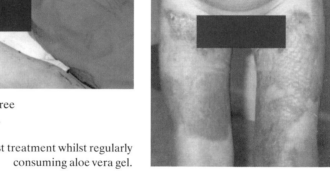

Post treatment whilst regularly consuming aloe vera gel.

Case Study - Burns

In January 1997 our two-year-old daughter caught fire from an unprotected gas flame. The burns were extensive, covering 14% of her body, mainly the inside of both legs, thighs and stomach. She was assessed at Warwick Hospital and transferred to the Special Burns Unit at Selly Oak Hosptial in Birmingham.

The treatment for full thickness burns at that time was to prick the large blisters which had quickly formed, give her morphine and antibiotics, and put her on a saline drip. The skin was left exposed and she was placed in an isolation room for several days under a large drying unit, which beamed hot air over the skin.

Finally, after several days, her burns were covered and bandaged, and the process of healing began.

Having been a family that ate a whole food, mainly organic diet with a strong belief in homeopathic and herbal remedies, I was horrified to see the amount of drugs which were required to sedate her and keep her free from infection, to say nothing of the blood packs which she required each time a new skin graft was performed (eight altogether).

The consultants and staff would not let us apply anything topically to aid the healing process, so I began to make phone calls to contacts in the natural health field. Several mentioned aloe vera gel, something she could drink rather than apply, so we began to add the gel to our daughter's drinks, two to three times daily.

There was then a period of almost six weeks when the burn sites were dressed and bandaged and the outer bandages were being changed every couple of days. We continued with the gel.

At the end of this time, we were told that our daughter would probably need to be sedated with Ketamine to make removal of the complete dressings possible. The sites would be very sore, sticky and extremely painful. The innermost dressing would have adhered to the sticky exudates and would be very difficult to remove. We prepared ourselves for the worst. As a family who had never even used Paracetamol before this event, I was loath to allow the doctors to administer Ketamine.

The outer bandages were removed and, as my daughter stood up to back away from this latest intrusion to her body, the inner bandages slipped down her legs revealing dry, pink, smooth scar tissue. There was very little pain.

The atmosphere in that room was amazing. The registrar was called, followed by the consultant, then another consultant. No one could believe that my daughter's third degree burns, followed by numerous skin grafts could have healed so quickly.

'How have you done this?' we were asked incredulously. Of course we were still shocked at the fact that our daughter was scarred; being involved with a burns patient is a slow dawning of realisation that this is something that we would live with forever. However, I have to say that we were delighted with the reaction of the staff. 'aloe vera gel!' I said. The looks that passed between the nurses spoke volumes. 'No seriously,' I said. 'We have been giving her 2 to 3 fl ozs every day. Now the bandages are off, can we put it on her skin too?'

Normally, at this stage, the burn site would be re-dressed and re-bandaged, in preparation for a further look two weeks down the line, but we were able to leave the site uncovered and start topical application immediately.

Five years on, we still apply Aloe Vera. The gel is now drunk by all of us. We are rarely ill and, compared to other children, both my daughters have only had one day off each from school. The consultants are very pleased with our progress, but we shall always be the aloe bunch from Leamington Spa.

Carrie Holmes

FUNGAL SKIN INFECTIONS

These are often difficult to treat and, if a topical Aloe Vera product is used, it must contain a high percentage of Aloe Vera, not less than around 60% stabilised aloe vera gel.

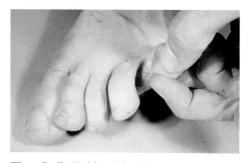

The creme should be applied after washing and thoroughly drying the area, as most fungicidal yeasts that

Tinea Pedis (Athlete's foot).

colonise human skin need a moist environment to survive.

VIRAL SKIN INFECTIONS

I have found two common viral skin infections that respond to Aloe Vera. These are Shingles (Herpes Zoster), and Molluscum Contagiosum, a tiresome condition that affects children. In the case of Shingles, the rash must be dealt with in the early stages and, because of skin sensitivity, a water-based aloe spray is ideal, followed by a gelly or creme, when the skin becomes less painful. I am certain that the natural antiviral activity of the long chain polysaccharide in the gel plays an important part in the process if drunk in sufficient quantities. My own small survey of patients has shown that the length of the cycle of the rash is reduced.

LICHEN PLANUS

Although an uncommon disease and one whose cause is not understood, Lichen Planus, especially where the rash involves the mouth, is a miserable condition to have. The evidence here is purely anecdotal, but for oral Lichen Planus, a combination of an aloe based tooth gel, an aloe gargle and a topical gelly can considerably ease the discomfort.

When the rash appears on the body, a strong topical product alleviates the itching and makes life more pleasant before it will hopefully spontaneously be resolved.

CHRONIC ULCERS & BED SORES

These wounds are notoriously difficult to heal because the blood supply to the site is poor and the wounds are also prone to infection, which hampers the healing process. The daily application of topical Aloe Vera after cleaning the wound, which must be kept in place, if necessary, with bandaging under an oc-clusive dressing, works in a good proportion of cases. Drinking Aloe Vera in tandem with the topical treatment will also improve the chances of success.

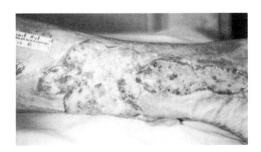

Infected chronic venous leg ulcer.

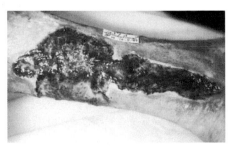

After 3 months of daily Aloe Vera dressings. Note the absence of infection.

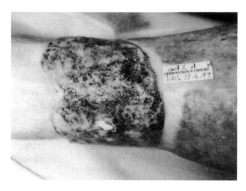
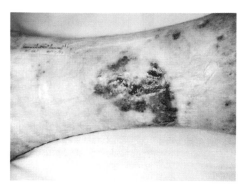

Chronic leg ulcer in a diabetic.   After 8 weeks on topical and oral Aloe Vera.

Case Study - Leg Ulcer

In 1998 I developed a pressure blister on the ball of my left foot, which soon became ulcerated. Having previously treated three similar ulcers successfully with aloe vera gelly, I wasn't too alarmed. However, within one week, scepticaemia set in and I was admitted to hospital, where a cocktail of antibiotics was given intravenously for the next four weeks. When it became obvious that there was no improvement, I was admitted to surgery. A trench was cut from between my first and second toe, to my ankle and the length of the top of my foot as, by now, abscesses and ulcers had formed along the length of the poison's track. I was discharged after five and a half weeks and, despite my request that aloe be used to treat the surgical wounds, they were treated with iodine.

Several months later, a fresh abcess was found between the first and second toes. I was told that the second toe would have to 'come off' after X rays had revealed Osteomyelitis. Surgery was scheduled four days after but, when no bed was available, the operation was postponed for six days.

In the meantime I went back into action. I took three fluid ounces of aloe vera gel every three hours, backed up with eight propolis tablets daily, taken in twos at mealtimes and last thing at night.

When the surgeon came to debride the new abcess, he could find no trace of the bacteria which had been attacking the bone, and so had no reason to amputate.

After this, both consultant and surgeon consented to my request to use aloe. From that time the wound was initially washed with aloe activator, then packed with aloe propolis creme, with a topping of aloe gelly to enhance absorption. The foot was then protected with a gauze dressing and bandage.

Subsequently, I continued to take propolis tablets – but only four a day - and although it was a long process, healing progressed well, and I was left with little scarring, despite the initial doubts of the consultant. Doctors and nurses were also impressed with the healing power of aloe.

Sally Barclay

ASTHMA

Asthma is due to an inflammation of the lining of the small tubes, or bronchioles, in the lungs. This causes them to narrow from the swelling, leading to the typical wheeze as the air passes through the narrowed passages. Associated with this inflammation there is often spasm of the muscle surrounding these passages, worsening the problem. There are many trigger factors associated with an attack. Common examples are allergy, infection, stress, physical exertion and changes in the ambient temperature. Attacks can be mild and short-lived or prolonged and life threatening. By drinking Aloe Vera on a regular basis, attacks can be reduced in frequency and severity due to its anti-inflammatory effect. If combined with another safe herb, Gingko Biloba, the smooth muscle around the bronchioles will relax, both actions leading to widening of the airways and easier breathing. Some sufferers may still need a 'puffer' for use in an attack, but my experience is that its use will be reduced.

Case Study - Asthma

My daughter was diagnosed with Asthma when she was three years old, after a severe attack. Luckily, her father has asthma and so he was quickly able to recognise the symptoms and get her the correct treatment. Having never dealt with asthma before, especially in a child, I was truly horrified to watch my daughter suffering, knowing that there was nothing I could do to help her or prevent it. As the years went on, my daughter was diagnosed with only mild asthma, suffering an attack once every month or so, or when she became ill, which in turn would invariably turn into a chest infection, thus triggering an asthma attack.

In March 2002, my whole family had been using its Aloe Vera products. My daughter, in particular, started taking an aloe drink with peaches which she calls her 'Happy Juice'. In the four months since starting the gel, she has only had one attack and has been able to reduce the number of times she needs to use her inhaler. She only takes ½ fl oz (15ml) of the gel a day but it seems to do the trick.

Justine King

THE DIGESTIVE TRACT

Epithelial tissue lines the whole of the digestive tract so, in principle, any problem from mouth ulcers, peptic ulcers in the stomach and duodenum, to Crohn's Disease, Diverticulitis or even Ulcerative Colitis can be helped by drinking Aloe Vera.

With all types of inflammatory bowel disease, I suggest that Aloe Vera is only started when the disease is in remission and stable and, even then, only a small amount, about 30mls per day, is used. I say this because for the first few days the condition can get a little worse before it gets better, so I always warn people that "it may stir them up a bit", producing a little pain with a looser stool. If the 30mls is well tolerated, the amount can be doubled at weekly intervals until a satisfactory amount is reached, usually somewhere between 100-200mls per day. A recent British clinical trial has shown that Aloe Vera is definitely superior to placebo in moderate ulcerative colitis, so I feel it is well worth trying.

IRRITABLE BOWEL SYNDROME (IBS)

Where there is normal bowel function, the famous nutritionist, Jeffrey Bland, has shown that Aloe Vera produces several effects when drunk on a daily basis:

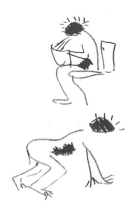

- It speeds up the transit time of the gut contents.
- As a result the stool becomes softer as it contains more water.
- Protein absorption is increased.
- Gut flora is regulated, especially where there is an overgrowth of the yeast Candida.

Perhaps it is one or all of these actions that bring about

A self portrait of an IBS sufferer showing her abdominal pain and mental stress.

GOOD HEALTH

The cactus drink that may help cure millions

Why irritable bowel sufferers swear by their daily dose of aloe vera juice

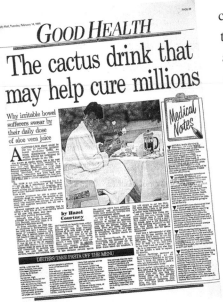

by Hazel Courtney

DIETERS TAKE PASTA OFF THE MENU

considerable improvement for the sufferers of this functional bowel problem that affects about 1 in 5 people in the western industrialised world at some time in their life.

Most people who suffer from it only do so mildly and rarely bother consulting their doctor about it. On the other hand, some people get it so severely that they can become prisoners in their own homes. They can never be far from a loo and dread the prospect of being caught short and having an accident. These people often experience explosive, sudden diarrhoea after a bout of colicky pain.

It is accepted that there is a stress element to this condition. However, apart from Aloe Vera's known ability to regulate and smooth out the gut's peristaltic movements, thereby reducing the pain and regulating the bowel habit, I believe it also has a calming effect on the mood, through its ability to balance the immune system and provide a greater sense of well being. Professionally, Aloe Vera is my first line treatment for IBS and I can claim about an 80% response rate.

Case Study - IBS

I have suffered from IBS for several years. Initially, I could not understand what was wrong with me. I had continual indigestion and always felt bloated, as though I was over-eating at every meal. Finally, I could not stand the discomfort any more and went to see my GP who put me on various anti-spasmodic drugs. However, although they kept the symptoms under control, I continued to have flare-ups.

I began taking aloe vera gel in August 2001 and, even after the second bottle, I could definitely feel an improvement. Since then I have not had any symptoms and I can eat anything I like. It is fantastic to be able to take a completely natural product instead of prescription drugs, which can produce awful side effects.

Originally, when introduced to a network level marketing company, I was interested in the powers of Aloe Vera and how natural products could play a part in improving the quality of life. At that stage, I didn't realise how powerful Aloe Vera was but am now totally convinced and will use it for the rest of my life.

Sue Rowbotham

ARTHRITIS

There are many different types of arthritis, but these can roughly be divided into two groups; those that involve an autoimmune process, a disorder of the immune system, where the body attacks itself, such as rheumatoid arthritis, psoriatic arthritis and the arthritis associated with systemic lupus and the other main group resulting from wear and tear, such as osteoarthritis.

Aloe Vera can help all forms of arthritis because of its natural anti-inflammatory and painkilling actions. This is particularly so in the types resulting from an immune disorder and in these cases there is an additional benefit resulting from the immuno-modulatory effect of the polysaccharide acemannan. When trying to help patients in this group, I usually recommend that Aloe Vera be given together with other natural anti-inflammatory substances containing Omega-3

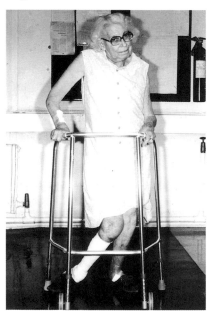

fatty acids. The two different types of anti-inflammatory action combine well and can reduce pain and stiffness, which in turn improves mobility.

Where there is wear and tear, such as in osteoarthritis, which affects many people to some extent over the age of 50, the anti-

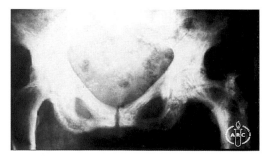

A severe case of osteoarthritis showing the characteristic deformities.

X-ray of a pelvis showing marked osteoarthritis of both hips.

inflammatory and painkilling effects of Aloe Vera can still be important in reducing symptoms. However, in this case, prevention is particularly important, especially in those groups of people that are more likely to develop the condition. These include females more so than males, serious athletes, the overweight and those involved in certain jobs such as heavy manual work.

I believe that anyone in the 'at risk' groups would benefit from taking Aloe Vera, possibly after the age of 40. However, in order to get the best results, combining it with other natural substances that form the basis of cartilage will prove most effective. These substances are glucosamine, chondroitin and methylsulphonyl methane (MSM). After the age of 40, people do not produce cartilage as effectively as when they were younger, so as joint cartilage is worn away during the day to day process of living, it's not replaced as efficiently and gradually becomes thinner. Eventually, it is so worn away that bone rubs against bone and a desperate situation ensues. By supplementing with the substances I've mentioned, the body's ability to make its own cartilage improves. I often use the analogy of a skyscraper being built. First the framework is established, represented by the glucosamine; then the gaps are filled with bricks or glass or other materials, which can be thought of as the chondroitin. They need to work together to get the best results, and are even better if MSM is also added. This natural anti-inflammatory organic sulphur compound which is already present in every cell in the body is vital for cartilage formation. The other process that happens over the years with osteoarthritis is that the fluid in the joint (synovial fluid) becomes thinner. Like oil in an engine, it needs to be of a certain thickness or viscosity to protect the moving parts. The same applies to the process within a joint. Chondroitin is what helps maintain this viscosity. The principle remains the same; we are simply providing the body with the additional ingredients needed to make the end product, in this case cartilage.

As well as drinking Aloe Vera, topical cremes can be used to rub on particularly tender areas on or around the joint. Once again MSM is particularly useful as an anti-inflammatory that can penetrate the skin when mixed with Aloe Vera.

Case Study -

I have suffered from Ankylosing Spondylitis since 1981. This disease is a chronic inflammation of the joints, mostly in the spine. The more common symptoms are pain and reduced mobility. The pain became increasingly bad several years ago, especially at night, waking me whenever I turned over. The prescribed medication was also unable to deal with the pain as effectively as it had previously.

I enjoy a busy life, but two of my most favourite activities involve considerable joint movement. I had just joined a brass band and was finding that blowing my instrument caused increased pain in my rib joints. I had also returned to the gym after a break of 18 months to recommence a health and fitness programme, only to find that there were several exercises that I had to avoid in order to prevent intense pain during subsequent days.

In March 2002, I began to drink aloe vera gel and from April changed to a drink containing aloe vera gel with glucosamine and chondroitin, increasing the amount from 60mls to 120mls daily. Within a few days, and ever since, I have been pain free during the day and, more importantly, at night as well.

I can now enjoy a good music session without pain, either whilst playing or subsequently. As for the gym, the levels of workout I can do have also been extended far beyond my dreams. I've strengthened and gained stamina and I feel great. My goal for this season...tennis!

Ruth Bricknell

LUPUS

Lupus is another auto-immune disease and is much commoner in women, especially of West Indian origin. Ninety five per cent of sufferers get muscle and joint problems and about 80% of these also develop skin rashes. The disease can also effect the nervous system, the kidneys, the respiratory system and the blood, so it can include many symptoms.

There is now a considerable amount of anecdotal evidence that sufferers have benefitted from taking aloe vera gel. I am sure that this is an effect of the polysaccharides helping to balance the immune system making it less likely to turn on its own tissues. I have known of a few cases where these people have been able to stop taking conventional medication usually in the form of steroids.

Case Study - Lupus

My wife, Brenda, became ill almost 19 years ago and, after eight years of visits to Harley Steet, was diagnosed with Lupus. She was subsequently prescribed various medications, including 20 mgs of steroids per day.

However, over the years, Brenda's condition grew steadily worse and, in October 1994, she was taking as many as 10 Paracetamol tablets for pain relief and between 45 and 50 mgs of steroids each day. The side effects of all this medication included excessive hair loss, brittle nails, irritable bowel, thinning of skin tissue, excessive weight gain, to name but a few. She was unable to participate in many of her previous pastimes and felt that life was barely worth living.

During October 1994, a friend who was a distributor of a muti level marketing company suggested that since she had absolutely nothing to lose, she might as well try a course of Aloe Vera. So she began and, within three months her health had already shown signs of improvement to the extent that she was able to reduce her usual medication.

She then doubled her intake of Aloe Vera and, by the end of February 1995 had halved her daily intake of medication. She also began to enjoy a better lifestyle, including recreational activities which had long been denied her.

Now, Brenda has stopped losing her hair and she also sports a beautiful set of nails; she has lost half a stone in weight and has been able to reduce her daily intake of medication to two Paracetamol and 5mgs of steroids. Most importantly, she feels healthy and active once again.

Frank Short

ADDITIONAL TREATMENTS. Other beneficial complementary therapies, which can be used in conjunction with Aloe Vera, can include acupuncture, often used very successfully with Chinese herbal medicine, homeopathy, aromatherapy, and naturopathy, where adding and eliminating certain foods from the diet, most commonly dairy products and wheat, can have very positive effects.

Other conditions can also be helped by Aloe Vera, either used topically or taken internally. These include:

Colitis
Crohn's Disease
Diverticulitis
Stomach Ulcers
Burns
Cold Sores
Diabetes
Gingevitis as well as Sensitive Teeth and Gums

Case Study – Stomach Ulcer

I've had a stomach ulcer, which became a lesion, for many years. Mostly, it was controlled with homeopathic or herbal remedies until several years ago, when it became worse, and I was frequently resorting to strong painkillers. I also began to see a direct link between stress levels at work (I'm a full-time teacher) and these attacks.

I came across an Aloe Vera drink at the same time that I was considering seeing a conventional doctor, when my stomach discomfort started to regularly prevent me from sleeping.

One day I came home from work with an unusually burning flare-up. Being new to the idea of drinking Aloe Vera, I was pretty sceptical about its effectiveness but, since the herbs and homeopathy weren't helping, it was worth a try. Almost immediately, I could feel the soothing benefits of the aloe as it came into contact with my stomach. It seemed to work as an extraordinary antacid, which counteracted the inflammation. I only had to increase the dose in order to completely overwhelm the burning sensations and then there was just this marvellous feeling of pain relief.

I subsequently had three or four similar episodes like this and it was a great comfort to know that a pharmaceutical-free pain relief was so quick and easy to obtain. Now, I only need to take a small amount daily as a maintenance dose and I haven't had a severe flare up for some time. My digestive system feels generally better too and not so prone to acidity.

Julie Harper

Case Study - Teeth & Gums

I have very strong teeth and had no cavities in over 30 years. I have used a well known toothpaste all my life and, I was slightly apprehensive about trying something different. They say that people with good teeth can have gum problems later in life. This proved to be true with my mother who has had gum surgery twice. I was keen to prevent this for myself. Although I have strong teeth, I do get a lot of plaque build-up, despite daily flossing.

When I visited my dentist after six months of using a toothgel containing Aloe Vera and bee propolis, I was very excited by his comment during the examination that my plaque build-up was significantly reduced and my gums were healthy with no bleeding at all. The added bonus is that my breath is fresher for longer during the day.

Lisa Hughes

Case Study - Cold Sores

Even as a child I was always susceptible to herpes simplex (cold sores). I was told it was lying dormant in my bloodstream and that stress, or exposure to certain weather conditions, would cause it to erupt.

Sadly, I proved that on my first skiing trip 22 years ago. Subsequently each year I have had my holidays seriously scarred by a disfigured face and distressing pain. Imagine being offered spaghetti Tabasco with your lips literally four times their size and blisters surrounding the mouth from nostrils to chin. On returning from holidays various people, seeing these cracking blisters, have assumed a car crash or something similar, so bad was my face.

My doctor abandoned me after prescribing Uvistat and then Herpid. He said: 'Give up skiing – stay indoors!' I changed doctors. A more sympathetic doctor prescribed Zovirax long before it was available over the counter, but it didn't work and I suffered minor side effects – a dry throat and flaky skin. Italian doctors gave me daily injections of goodness knows what in my buttock.

At last, in 1994, armed only with aloe vera gel, aloe lips, aloe sunscreen and aloe soap, I went skiing. We experienced eight days of skiing incorporating all weathers – sun, wind, blizzards. I now needed no more proof. Each day after that, I woke with beautiful lips thanks to these great products.

Vivien Ellis

Case Study - Colitis

In 1984, at the age of 32, I was diagnosed with Ulcerative Colitis. The symptoms were loss of blood and mucus due to ulceration of the large bowel and rectum, resulting in a lack of control of my bodily functions. In addition, I had painful arthritis in my joints. These symptoms combined with a complete lack of energy and mental anguish, made life a complete misery.

I was soon warned that the ulceration could develop into cancer and, with our first child due within a month, I had no choice other than to have the operation available to relieve my condition and save my life. It is called an ileostomy, which means that the large bowel is removed, the stomach is connected to the small bowel (the ileum) and a part of the ileum is taken outside the body and formed into a spout to pass the body's waste into a replaceable receptacle. The rectum is removed and the aperture sewn up. It was possible to have a 'reversal' operation where a pouch is cut out of the abdomen to partially take the place of the large bowel but, in my case, my illness had advanced too seriously.

However, after three operations, I suffered from arthritis, many severe gastric upsets, severe cramps, backache, sinusitis, chest infections, body overheating, together with generally very poor health and lack of energy. Despite spending hundreds of pounds on alternative medicine, including acupuncture, no permanent relief was obtained.

In 1995, I was introduced to an Aloe Vera juice drink, which gave me a little relief. Then I was introduced to an American Aloe Vera drinking gel and, within a very short period, I experienced a dramatic improvement in my overall health and wellbeing. All the above ailments are now gone or significantly improved and my life has been transformed. I can now work, play with my sons and have a social life.

Stephen Hatch

Case Study - Diabetes

In 2001, at the age of 10, my son Adam was diagnosed with diabetes. After the initial shock wore off we were shown how to monitor his blood sugar levels.

As expected, at first they were erratic. Doctors tried for a long time to stabilise them between five and 10, altering his insulin on an almost daily basis. No matter what was tried – more or less insulin – the levels were either too high or far too low. Eventually the doctors decided on the level of insulin to be given even though his blood sugar level was still high (12-17). It was finally accepted that his levels would be high, averaging out at 15, and would be unlikely to change.

Some time later we tried a drink containing aloe vera gel with glucosamine and chondroitin. Adam thought it tasted horrible but persevered, as he hoped it would do him good. Within a few days his blood sugar levels started to fall. We did not know why this was but we were pleased. Adam carried on drinking the gel but he was happier when we changed to a drink containing Aloe Vera, cranberries and apple.

Now, his blood sugar levels are stablised at an average of eight. It can only be due to the aloe vera gel since nothing else was changed in his routine.

Jill Pitcher

Case Study - Crohn's Disease

I was diagnosed as having Crohn's Disease in 1982. To anyone who may not know, Crohn's Disease is a severe disorder of the stomach and bowel. For me it caused such disabling bouts of severe diarrhoea and stomach cramping, that I was unable to work or function properly from day to day. Both my social and working lives had to be planned and reorganised daily, depending on my condition.

Serious dietary changes over eight years failed to help. These changes varied, from including and excluding various foods, including vegetables and 'starch', to alcohol and common beverages. Time passed, with two operations and several changes of medication, which caused unpleasant side effects and worsened my conditions.

Left in medical limbo, and despite my scepticism, I turned to a multi level marketing company that made a product containing Aloe Vera, cranberries and apple in desperation. I can now laugh and sing out loud; I can work effortlessly and I no longer have to plan around my condition. In a word,

I have returned to pre-1984 when my stomach and bowels were normal and can eat things I never thought possible. It took me only three months of taking two fluid ounces three times a day to achieve this wonderful feeling, although I did get positive results after just three weeks.

Gerard Roache

Case Study- Diverticulitis

I have suffered from Diverticulitis for many years and I have had to go to my local hospital on several occasions. It was so bad that I was unable to take on a full-time job as I had the embarrassment of constantly running to the toilet. I was on medication and was unable to go on holiday without it.

I was introduced to a drink containing Aloe Vera, cranberries and apple and all I can say is that I feel absolutely great. I am now working full-time at our local post office and my family is extremely relieved that I can now live a normal life.

Yvonne Dudley

The Case Study reports contained herein are the actual testimonials provided by the person or persons reflected in each report. In most instances, those people giving testimonials were so impressed with the products that they became distributors for the company marketing the products. The testimonials reflect the experiences of the individuals and are anecdotal. They are not based upon any clinical study and may be atypical. They are reproduced here for the reader for educational purposes because they are consistent with the results that I have observed in my practice. I believe that they clearly indicate further research is warranted.

A Naturopathic View

Aloe Vera might be able to alleviate and even cure a variety of ills but, without some input in other areas, money spent on either the juice or the gel could be wasted and the healing process hindered.

It's all very well waxing the car and changing the wipers, but using a poor grade oil or fuel, or driving badly, will eventually take its toll.

In the same way, we need to take care of our bodies, particularly these days when the stresses and strains that affect it are increasing, and the build-up of pollutants in our atmosphere is increasing the incidences of allergies and intolerances.

The organic farming movement is growing rapidly which, from the point of view of taste, is certainly to be encouraged. However, I would personally much rather eat non-organically grown fresh food than organic food that has been chilled, stored and then displayed for several days on the shelves of one of our main supermarkets. Fruit and vegetables in particular need to be eaten within a few days, and preferably a few hours, of harvesting before the natural degradation process starts and the potency of the vitamins, minerals and trace elements is lost. These are vital to the well being of our enzyme systems and our subsequent health.

Several authorities think that the rise in cancer rates is due to increased exposure to the harmful free radicals which emanate from the many forms of pollution that affect us, combined with our inability to fight them. Free radicals cause the highly destructive oxidative damage and in order to combat this threat, we need to be armed with anti-oxidants, not only using our naturally occurring antioxidant enzymes, but also the antioxidants we ingest in our food, for example vitamins A, C & E, and minerals such as Selenium and Zinc and the bioflavonoids.

Take a look at cancer of the prostate gland. Its incidence is now fast approaching that of cancer of the breast in women and there is strong evidence that a major factor may simply be selenium deficiency. Selenium is the most powerful mineral antioxidant and is often lacking in food because it is not present in sufficient quantities in the soil.

For that reason, attention paid to diet, exercise and relaxation techniques can work wonders in themselves. A number of inflammatory and other illnesses can be caused and exacerbated by lack of attention to lifestyle, and when this is the case, any positive effects of using Aloe Vera may well be lessened.

For some people, the effort involved in looking after their body is unacceptable; they just can't be bothered. It's maybe only later in life that they start counting the cost of any earlier neglect or excess. Before that happens, a simple healthy diet, together with some form of regular exercise, can easily become a way of life, especially when it begins to show a positive effect.

DIET

The body is composed entirely of molecules derived from food. In a lifetime you will consume around 100 tons of the stuff which, during the digestion process, is broken down by enzyme-rich secretions in the digestive tract, produced at a rate of about 10 litres a day. So it's obvious that the role of diet, as well as exercise, is a vital one.

Poor nutrition ultimately means poor health in one form or another. Nor can you escape your background. Poor nutrition experienced over generations is recorded and expressed genetically as various strengths and weaknesses in the body. So anything positive you can do now will not only store up potential good health for the future but will also help to repair negative states from the past. You will have more resistance to disease and will experience increased health and vitality.

A healthy programme might include the following:

Exercise, both aerobic and for relaxation
Eating plenty of complex carbohydrates, i.e. grains, pulses, fruits and vegetables
Eating plenty of nuts, seeds and yellow and green leafy vegetables
Limiting intake of animal protein, especially red meat, an excess of which is linked to cancer of the colon.

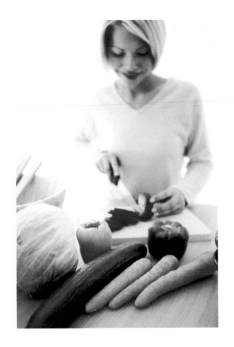
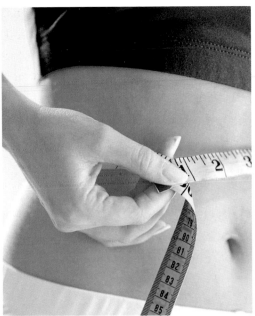

Cutting down on salt and processed foods

Cutting down on sugar

Avoiding fried and fatty foods (excluding stir fries)

Reduction of dairy intake

Cutting down on alcohol and caffeine

Stopping smoking

At times of stress or illness, taking a good multivitamin and mineral supplement, and raising your intake of Vitamin C can also be a useful boost for the immune system.

The role of diet can also play a part in helping to control certain conditions like eczema and psoriasis, which are often exacerbated by spicy food, dairy products, citrus fruits, alcoholic drinks, coffee and fry-ups.

EXERCISE

It's official, exercise not only helps keep you healthy but also helps you unwind and recharges your batteries.

For some people, exercise is an essential and enjoyable part of their lives. For others even walking to the postbox to post a letter is a huge effort. They'd rather hop in a car than use their own motive power any day. This is all very well when you're in the first flush of youth, but eventually lack of good aerobic activity will not only impair your health, but also your state of well-being.

The reasons why exercise makes you feel good is that it triggers the release of endorphins, the chemicals in the brain that make you generally feel happier, calmer and more clear-headed.

It's important to choose some form of exercise which suits you. It's no good jogging or swimming if you get no pleasure from either, especially if you have a dodgy knee joint or can't swim. This could add to any stress you might already be under – and you might drown!!.

Choose something you will enjoy for half an hour at least three times a week. It is much better to do a little exercise regularly than make a marathon effort just once in a while, and possibly have a heart attack or strain yourself.

Whatever form of exercise you choose, it should raise your pulse rate and leave you a little breathless immediately after it. So, it's important to go easy on yourself at the beginning, building up slowly and gently. Yoga or Pilates are good for improving flexibility, as well as for relaxation; weight training is ideal for strength; and brisk walking or swimming helps with endurance.

Physical activities that free the mind are also very therapeutic, like long-

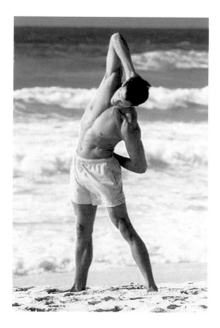 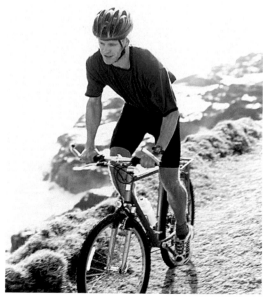

distance walking, cycling or swimming. You can also try the ancient Chinese art of T'ai Chi, a form of moving meditation and if you don't know how to get started on your own, exercise with a friend or join a gym or club to get you going and keep you motivated.

It's ideal to include more than one type of exercise in your programme. Variety is the spice of life after all and, as well as holding your interest, it will work out different parts of your body.

Once you start exercising, it's important to remember to use the right fuel and that means eating the right foods and eliminating junk food from your diet, although the odd piece of cake or a sweet once in a while can still be included. There's no need to make sacrifices or go without your dearest edible pleasures completely. You may just find you don't crave them as much as you did once you start feeling healthier.

And DO stop smoking. Smoking not only ultimately creates havoc with your internal organs but also damages the skin, thus speeding up the ageing process and without the demon weed, you'll be able to get up that hill and swim that lap without gasping for breath.

RELAXATION

Exercise will help you to unwind and relax, but if you're especially tense, a spot of T'ai chi or yoga will 'sooth the savage breast' as well as relax tense muscles. Meditation – and there are various simple techniques – is not only relaxing but, carried out over a period of time, will help encourage a more positive state of mind, boost the immune system, and counteract the negative effects of stress. This can be very helpful with illnesses such as asthma, and with inflammatory skin conditions.

So whilst Aloe Vera can play a positive part in the alleviation and even elimination of certain conditions, its path can only be positively smoothed by attention to how you live your life and treat your body. It's all part of the picture of health.

Animals &
ALOE VERA

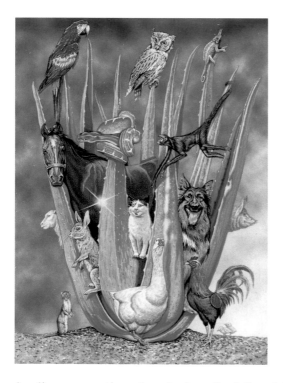

With vets' bills apparently escalating, it is hardly surprising that farmers, pet owners and those involved with horses, are anxious to help treat the animals in their care, whenever possible, by using effective first aid measures. Many people who take care of animals do not wish to use powerful drugs because of the various and sometimes unpleasant side effects they can cause. Nor do they wish to subject their beloved animals to chemicals unless absolutely necessary.

This is where Aloe Vera can be a huge benefit because of its proven healing properties, already described. In addition, Aloe Vera taken orally is a natural anti-pruritic and reduces the itching that occurs in many skin complaints, especially allergic dermatitis, because it inhibits the body's ability to produce histamine. Trying to prevent animals from scratching and exacerbating an existing condition, can be extremely difficult and often requires animals to wear futuristic looking devices as a preventative measure.

With the wide range of good Aloe Vera products now available, animal custodians, both commercial and domestic, can often intervene before an appointment with the veterinary surgeon becomes necessary, to reduce the symptoms, initiate healing and even prevent infection.

A colleague of mine, and one of the UK's leading equine vets, David Urch, is the greatest advocate of Aloe Vera in practice. His book 'Aloe Vera – Nature's Gift' has to be the definitive work on the various veterinary applications of Aloe Vera. Because of this, I will not attempt to describe in detail the various conditions that Aloe Vera can benefit. For those interested in this aspect of Aloe, his book is therefore a must, and is listed in the Further Reading section of the book.

Topical products such as Aloe Vera spray, soap, gel and propolis creme, can be used to treat various inflammatory skin conditions such as dermatitis, eczema and those where bacterial infection is present, such as abscesses, boils and infected insect bites. Fungal infections such as ringworm can also be helped, together with traumatic abrasions and ulceration from a badly fitting harness, for example. Various kinds of wounds, such as incised wounds from sharp objects, e.g. barbed wire, as well as ulcers and burns, will also heal much more quickly.

A good general regime would include:

- Removal of any foreign body or obvious cause, where possible.

- Cleanse the area using water or, where obviously contaminated, with Aloe Vera soap.

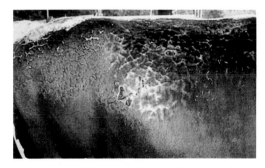

Cow severly burnt in an arson attack.

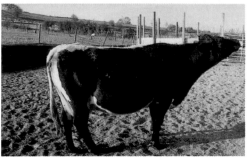

Several months later the wounds have completely healed.

- Expose the area by removing any matted hair around the wound site.

- Use an Aloe Vera spray on the wound and surrounding area and follow up with an application of aloe vera gelly.

Initially, the gel should be applied quite often, say four to six times each day. The frequency can then be reduced as the wound becomes clean and starts to show newly healing or "granulation" tissue.

It is generally found that, with the Aloe Vera healing process, not only will there be minimal scar formation but also, when new fur or hair appears, the re-growth will be the original colour rather than white, as is often the case. This is a major plus when show animals are affected.

As with the human healing process, all the elements necessary to produce healthy skin cells are supplied to an area via the bloodstream. This can be precipitated by adding aloe vera gel to animal feed. This can be problematic with cats, which are notoriously fussy and may not like the taste. One solution is to paint it on their fur, which they will soon lick clean.

Using aloe internally is, I believe, one of the most efficacious ways to promote healing. In fact, an animal does not need to have a problem or to be ill in order to benefit from Aloe Vera. It can also be used as a general tonic to improve the quality of hair, fur, feather and skin.

Remember that skin appendages, like hair, horns and claws, are all epithelial tissue. All have been shown to grow faster and more luxuriantly under the influence of aloe. I know two people, one of whom breeds racing pigeons and the other who shows pet rats, who attribute much of their protegees' success to the addition of aloe vera gel to their food.

In order to demonstrate aloe's effect on epithelial tissue in animals, David Urch organised a clinical trial to measure the rate of growth of horses' hooves. Half the horses in the study received standard fodder, whilst the other half had aloe vera gel added daily to their food. At the end of the trial, the aloe-treated horses' hooves had grown considerably faster than the control group. If it can have such a positive effect on hooves, surely there are distinct possibilities for human hair and nails. It may be of interest to note that since using aloe regularly, I have had to visit the barber more often than I used to; it's a shame that Aloe Vera hasn't done more to restore the colour! – I am quite grey.

The table below will give you an idea of the amounts to use

ANIMAL	TREATMENT DOSE PER DAY	MAINTENANCE & GENERAL TONIC
Hamsters, Mice, Gerbils (50-100g)	2mls	½ ml
Rats, Pigeons, Guinea Pigs, Chinchillas, Ferrets Rabbits (400g-2kg)	4mls	1ml
Cats (5kg)	20mls	5mls
Dogs (30kg)	60mls	15mls
Sheep, Pigs (150kg)	120mls	30mls
Cows (500kg)	250mls	60mls
Horses (500kg)	250mls	60mls

Aloe vera gel can also be added to the food or the drinking water.

Animals, like humans, are prone to viral infections, especially 'flu' like viruses. Whilst most fully recover, a small percentage go on to develop a post-viral fatigue syndrome similar to ME (Myalgic Encephalitis) which affects humans. Like humans, animals become lethargic and tire easily when exercising. With horses, this condition can be particularly pronounced and debilitating. There has been a marked lack of success with conventional treatment, with the result that many of these animals are unable to return to their previous activities such as racing, dressage or eventing.

Unlike humans, horses affected by this condition also develop changes in the blood, with white blood cell counts sometimes dropping to almost fatal levels. Another equine vet, Peter Green, whose stables were affected by 'flu' and subsequent post-viral lethargy in 14 of his animals, wrote an article in the Veterinary Times. It described his use of aloe vera gel and his success in getting 11 out of the 14 horses back to their original strength and activities, something previously unheard of. Luckily, he took blood samples from all the horses before and after the aloe treatment. These showed that, as expected, prior to treatment, all the horses showed a reduced white cell count, but after treatment the improved horses showed a rise in the white cell count and a return to normal levels.

I am sure this activity is attributable to the immuno-modulating effect of the long chain sugar 'acemannan' derived from the mucilage layer of the Aloe Vera plant and found in the gel.

In the USA, Carrington Laboratories have extracted this sugar and developed it into a conventional drug, Carrisyn, which is licensed by the Food and Drugs Administration (FDA) to treat leukaemia in cats. Feline leukaemia is caused by a retro-virus and this cancer of the blood is now effectively treated by the aloe extract. The great retro-viral illness currently affecting mankind is AIDS, caused by HIV. I understand that a similar drug also developed by Carrington Laboratories is now being trialled by HIV sufferers.

The tables listed in this chapter are taken from David Urch's book, with his kind permission.

ALOE VERA
the Future

When I was introduced to Aloe Vera ten years ago, like the majority of other people in the UK, I had never heard of it. Since then, however, it has steadily increased in popularity and has now established itself as a marketing buzz word ingredient. It has been added to an increasing variety of products and the 'with aloe' tag is commonplace. The problem is that the small quantities that are usually added are unlikely to produce any beneficial results.

Cosmetic firms, such as Clairol, have added it to shampoo, Revlon has added it to lipstick, and Gillette has included it in an after-shave product. Because of its soothing and moisturising effects it has been added to tissues for every body orifice! It has even been added to babies' nappies, latex examination gloves and women's tights. Quite why it has been added to the latter I just do not know. It also appears regularly in mouthwashes and gargles. Perhaps the ultimate accolade was when Persil made the decision to add it to their famous washing powder. Aloe Vera is now firmly established as an important and useful ingredient and is recognised as such by most of the buying public.

I am certain that cosmetic companies will continue to exploit the moisturising and anti-aging properties of Aloe Vera. However, for me, Aloe Vera's importance in the future lies in its clinical application. It has already been accepted by many of the more open-minded physicians and surgeons and is currently used at the Great Ormond Street Hospital for Sick Children in London to treat the rare and distressing blistering skin disease, Epidermolysis Bullosa. It has found favour in many other hospital departments that carry out skin procedures which can result in pain, bruising or even burning; for example, in post laser treatment for birth marks and following radiotherapy in the treatment of cancer.

We have already covered the usage of Aloe Vera in ancient beauty regimes. Today it is widely used as a topical application after leg waxing, the removal of superfluous hair or after the treatment of thread veins. The application of Aloe Vera following these procedures relieves pain and reduces swelling and inflammation.

In order to convince the medical fraternity of the clinical benefits of Aloe Vera, it has always been necessary to present the evidence in a form that it understands and accepts; usually this has to be the clinical trial.

Until recently, documented trials were regrettably not of the quality and precision that were likely to win over the sceptical, scientifically orientated doctor, especially with the current emphasis of evidence based medicine. Any overwhelming anecdotal evidence has largely been ignored by regular practitioners, but fortunately there are some who have given it a try. I know a handful of doctors, both in the National Health Service and in the private sector, who now regularly use aloe in their practices.

A small but significant early trial was carried out in 1985 by Dr Jeffrey Bland, a nutritionist at the Linus Pauling Institute of Science and Medicine in California. Bland studied the effect of Aloe Vera on the gastrointestinal function in healthy humans, involving ten volunteers in the study, five of each sex. The volunteers changed nothing in their lifestyle, but consumed two fluid ounces of Aloe Vera juice three times a day for seven consecutive days. Beforehand, the participants fasted overnight so that base line gastric secretion could be measured by a pH (level of acidity) sensitive capsule. After their gastric pH was measured, a morning stool and urine sample were collected. The object of the experiment was to see if aloe had any effects on these two functions. Dr Bland looked at urinary indican, which reflects the bowel bacterial conversion of the amino acid tryptophan, and therefore possible improved protein digestion and absorption, after Aloe Vera treatment. He also looked at stool specific gravity, gastric pH and bowel motility.

He found that, after one week on aloe, urinary indican levels were lowered, suggesting an increase in both protein breakdown and absorption. He also found stool specific gravity was reduced, with a faster movement of stool through the bowel. Both these findings indicated an increase in water in the stool, although no diarrhoea was reported. He also found the pH was normalised or buffered, meaning that Aloe Vera had acted as an alkalising agent.

He commented that Aloe Vera had helped to normalise stool bacterial cultures in six subjects, four of the six having previously had high yeast levels in their gut.

In discussing his findings, Jeffrey Bland said:

'The tolerance of the subjects to Aloe Vera juice supplementation was in general quite good. One person complained of gas and another of transient gut pain which, after continued supplementation throughout the week, diminished. The other eight subjects were asymptomatic with no diarrhoea, nausea, intestinal bloating or distress. Four of the subjects had noted improved bowel regularity, with greater gastrointestinal comfort after eating. Three indicated that they felt some enhancement of energy and a sense of well-being, although this could not be confirmed quantitatively'.

Personally, I am pleased to report that the first trial in which I became involved four years ago has now come to a conclusion. This was a trial using Aloe Vera drinking gel in the treatment of ulcerative colitis. It was carried out on 44 patients and was a truly randomised, double-blind, placebo controlled trial, using two major teaching hospitals, the Barts and the NHS Trust in East London and the John Radcliffe in Oxford. The lead physician was Professor David Rampton, whose conclusion at the end of the trial was:

"Oral Aloe Vera taken for four weeks produces a clinical response more often than with a placebo; it also improves histological disease activity and appears to be safe. These encouraging results suggest that further evaluation of the thera-peutic potential of aloe vera gel in inflammatory bowel disease is warranted."

I am now awaiting the results of an even bigger trial, which I helped set up in 2001, involving 200 patients using the same drinking gel in the treatment of irritable bowel syndrome (IBS). The trial is now nearing conclusion at the Morriston Hospital, part of the Welsh National Medical School in Swansea. This time, the trial is headed by the Professor of Surgery, John Baxter.

I think that Aloe Vera's future is now assured. It has established itself as an important supplement at a time when there is huge growth in complementary and alternative medicine. People, especially in the UK, are constantly being reminded that they should take responsibility for their own health and look after themselves by maintaining a healthy lifestyle, involving general fitness, a balanced diet and the avoidance of over-exposure to free radicals found in pollutants such as cigarette smoke, exhaust fumes and herbicides and pesticides.

In a society where cancer rates are rising, despite the fact that death rates are falling, one should follow the advice that Hipprocates gave when he said,

'let medicine be thy food and food be thy medicine'.

I believe our increased exposure to these free radicals could account for this increase in cancer. So, apart from avoiding them when we can, we need to protect ourselves from the oxidative damage that they cause and the only way we can do that is with anti-oxidants.

Despite the fact that we have to cope with free radicals produced by the metabolism or burning of our food to liberate energy, our bodies possess enzymes, the most important of which is nicknamed "SOD" (Super Oxide Dismutase) which can neutralise them. The important aspect is balance; if we have enough SOD or we don't produce too much free radical then all is well. It is only when the balance shifts that we run an increased risk of developing cancer.

The other important part of this process is the anti-oxidants that we find in our food, mostly from fruit and vegetables, especially dark green broad leaf vegetables such as cabbage and kale, and seed bearing vegetables, such as broccoli, legumes or beans. It has been said that we should eat five portions of vegetables and fruit per day, but latest American research now suggests that it should be nine portions, due to the deterioration in the quality of our food. There are increasingly less nutrients in the soil and therefore less in our food. Aloe Vera, however, tends to grow in areas which are rich in minerals and micro-nutrients and so, as our food gets worse, Aloe Vera is an important supplement.

It has also been said, by a famous Auryvedic physician that,

'if the diet is good then medicines are of no need, but if the diet is bad medicines are of no use'.

As with all Aloe Vera products, however, the final outcome depends upon two main considerations which are of paramount importance: the amount of Aloe Vera that is actually included in the product and the quality of the manufacturing process. It should be produced in such a way that there is minimal interference with the extract from the plant, i.e. there should be no overheating, minimal filtration and no concentration. Additives to stabilise and preserve the product should be naturally sourced rather than using man-made chemicals, so that the ultimate product is as near as possible to the natural plant extract.

I will leave it to Christopher Columbus, the fifteenth century explorer, to sum up. He said:

'Four vegetables are indispensable for the well-being of man: wheat, the grape, the olive and the aloe. The first nourishes him, the second raises his spirit, the third brings him harmony, and the fourth cures him'.

References

Bland, J.Effect of Orally Consumed Aloe Vera Juice on Gastrointestinal Fuction in Normal Humans. *Prevective Medicine, March/April 1985.*

Coates. B.C *The Silent Healer: Amodern Study of Aloe Vera.* Garland, Texas, 1979.

Danhof, I.E., McAnalley, B.H. Stablilised Aloe Vera-Effect on Human Skin Cells. *Drug and Cosmetic Inustry*, 133:52,54, 105-106 (1983).

Davis, R.H : Leitner, M.G. ; Russo, J.M. Aloe Vera, a Natural Aproach for Treating Wounds, Oedema and in Diabetes. *J. Am. Podiart. Med. Assoc.*, 78(2): 60-68 (1988).

Davis R,H.; Parker W.L.; Murdoch D.P. Aloe Vera as a Biologically Active Vehicle for Hydrocortisone Acetate. *J. Am. Podiart. Med. Assoc.*, 81(1): 1-9 (1991).

Davis, R.H.: Rosenthal, K.Y.: Cesario, L.R.; Rouw, G.A. Processed Aloe Vera Adminisered Topically Inhibits Inflamation. *J. Am. Podiatr. Med. Assoc.*, 79(8):395-97 (1989)

Davis, R.H.: Stewart, G.J.: Bregman, P. J. Aloe Vera and the Inflamed Synovial Pouch, Model. *J. Am. Podiatr. Med. Assoc.*, 82(3): 140-48 (1992).

Fujita, K.; Ho, S.: Teradaira, R.; Beppu, H. Properties of Carboxypeptidase from Aloe. *Biochemical Pharmacology*, 28: 1261-62 91979).

Fujita, K.; Teradaira , R. Nagatsu, T. Bradykinase Activity of Aloe Extract. *Biochemical Pharmacology*, 25:205 (1976)

Fulton, J.E. The Stimulation of Postdermabrasioon Wound Healing with Stabilised aloe vera gel Polyethylene Oxide Dressing. *J. Dermatol. Surg. Oncol.* 16(5):460-67 (1990).

Green. P. Aloe Vera Extracts in Equine Clinical Practice. *Vet. Times*, September 1996, p. 9.

Grindlay, D. : Reynolds, T. The Aloe Vera Phenomenon: Areview of the Properties and Modern Uses of the Leaf Parenchyma *Gel. J. Ethnopharmacol,* 16:117-51 (1986).

Heggars, J.P.: Kucukelesi, A.; Lisengarten, D. et al, Beneficial Effect of Aloe on Wound Healing in an Excisional Wound Model. *J. Alt. Complement. Med,.* 2(2):271-77 (1996).

Heggars, J.P.; Pelley, R.D.; Robson, M.C Beneficial Effects of Aloe in Wound Healing. *Phytother. Res.*, 7: 48-52 (1993).

Ito, S.; Teradaira, R; Beppu, H.; Obata, M.; Fujita, K.; Nagatsu, T. Biochemical Properties of Carboxypeptidase from Aloe aborescens Millei var. Natalensis Berger. *Phytother. Res.,* 7: 26 29 (1993).

Kahlon, J.B.; Kemp, M.C.; Carpenter, R.H.; McAnalley, B.H.; McDaniel, H.R.; Shannon, W.M. Inhibition of AIDS Virus Replication by Acemannan in vitro. *Mol. Biother,* 3: 127-35 (1991).

Kahlon, J.B.; Kemp, M.C. Yaweci, N.; Carpenter, R.H.; Shannon, W.M.; McAnalley, B.H. In vitro Evaluation of the Synergistic Antiviral Effects of Acemannan in Combination with Azidothymidine and Acyclovir. *Mol. Biother.*, 3: 214-23 (1991).

Langmead, L.; Feakins, R.M.; Goldthorpe, S.; Holt, H.; Tsironi, E.; De Silva, A.; Jewell, D.P.; Rampton, D.S.; Randomised double-blind, placebo-controlled trial of oral aloe vera gel for active ulcerative colitis. *Aliment Pharmacol Ther* 2004; 19:739-747.

Lorenzetti, L.J.; Salisbury, R.; Beal, J.L.; Baldwin, J.N. Bacteriostatic Property of Aloe Vera. *J. Pharm. Sci.,* 53: 1287 (1964).

McDaniel, H.R.; McAnalley, B.H. evaluation of Polymannoacetate (Carrisyn) in the Treatment of AIDS. *Clin. Res.*, 35: 483A (1987).

Marshall, G.D.; Gibbons, A.S.; Parnell, L.S. Human Cytokines Induced by Acemannan. *J. Allergy Clin. Immunol.*, 91: 295 (1993).

Obata, M.; Ibo, S.; beppu, H.; Fujita, K.; Nagatsu, T. Mechanism of Anti-inflammatory and Anti-thermal Burn Action of C Pase from Aloe aborescens Miller var. Natalensis Bergr in Rats and Mice. *Phytother. Res., 7* (Special Issue): 530-33 (1993).

Robson, M.C.; Heggers, J.P.; Hagstrom, W.J. Myth, Magic, Witchcraft, or Fact? Aloe Vera revisited. *J. Burn Care Rehab.*, 3:157-62 (1982).

Rowe, T.D.; Parks, L.M. A Phytochemical Study of Aloe Vera Leaf. *J. Am. Pharm. Assoc.*, 39: 262-65 (1939).

Saito, H. Purification of Active Substances in Aloe Vera arborescenes Miller and their Biological and Pharmacological Activity. *Phytother. Res.,* 7: 17-19 (1993). (Special Issue: Proceedings of the International Congress of Phytotherapy, 1991).

Sendelbach, L.E. A Review of the Toxicity and Carcinogenicity of Anthraquinone Derivatives. *Toxicology,* 57:227-40 (1989).

Sheets, M.A.; Under, B.A.; Gielleman, G.F.; Tizard, I.R. Studies of the Effect of Acemannan on Retrovirus Infections: Clinical Stabilisation of Feline Leukaemia Virus Infected Cats. *Mol Biother.*, 3:41-45 (1991).

Shelton, M.S. Aloe Vera, Its Chemical and Therapeutical Properties. *Internat. J. Dermatology,* 30:679-83 (1991).

Sims, R.M.; Zimmermann, E.R. Effect of Aloe Vera on Herpes Simplex and Herpes Virus (Strain Zoster). *Aloe Vera of America Archives. Stabilized Aloe Vera*, Vol.1, pp 237-38. 1971.

Sims, R.M.; Zimmermann, E.R. Report – The Effect of Aloe Vera on Mycotic Organisms (Fungi). *Aloe Vera of America Archives. Stabilized Aloe Vera*, Vol.1, pp 237-38. 1971.

Syed, T.; Ahmed A.; Holt, A.; Ahmad, S., et al. Management of Psoriasis with Aloe Vera Extract in a Hydrophilic Creme: a Placebo Controlled Double Blind Study. *Tropical Med. Internat. Health*, 1(4): 505-509 (1996).

Syed T.A.; Afsal M.; Ashfa Q.; Ahmad S.; Holt A.N.; Ahmad Ali S.; Ahmad S.H. Management of Genital Herpes in men with 0.5% Aloe Vera extract in a hydrophilic creme: a placebo controlled double blind study. Journal of Dermatological Treatment. 1997.8.99-102.

Teradaira, R.; Shimzato, M.; Beppu, H.; Fujita, K. Antigastric Ulcer Effects in Rats of Aloe arborescens Miller var. Natalensis Berger *Extract Phytother. Res.*, 7:534-36 (1993).

Udupa, S.L.; A.L.; Kulkarni, D.R. Anti-inflammotory and Wound Healing Properties of Aloe Vera. *Fitoterapia*, 65 (2):141-45 (1994).

Vogler,B.K.; Ernst E. Aloe Vera. A systematic review of its clinical effectiveness. British Journal of General Practice 1999, 49, 823-828.

Winters, W.D.; Immunoreactive Lectins in Leaf Gel from Aloe barbadensis Miller. *Phytother. Res.*, 7:23-25 (1993).

Winters, W.D.; Benavide, R.; Clouse, W.J. Effects of Aloe Extracts on Human Normal and Tumour Cells in vitro. *Econ. Bot.*, 35:89-95 (1981).

Glossary

Acemannan. A complex carbohydrate considered to be one of the many active ingredients found in aloe.

Raw Aloe Vera Gel. Naturally occurring, unprocessed, undiluted parenchymal tissue obtained from the decorticated leaves of Aloe Barbadensis Miller (Aloe Vera linné), to which no other material has been added.

Aloe Vera Gel. Naturally occurring, processed, undiluted parenchymal tissue obtained from the decorticated leaves of Aloe Barbadensis Miller.

100% Aloe Vera. Processed, preserved liquid derived from parenchymal tissue obtained from the decorticated leaves of Aloe Barbadensis Miller (Aloe Vera linné)

Whole Aloe Vera Gel. Aloe Vera Gel, which contains a minimum of 50% of the natural pulp found in raw Aloe Vera Gel.

Aloe Vera Latex. The bitter yellow liquid contained in the pericyclic tubules of the rind of Aloe Barbadensis Miller; the principal constituent of which is aloin.

Whole Leaf Aloe Vera. Whole leaf of the Aloe Barbadensis Miller, including the rind and internal portions of the plant.

Aloe USP. The dried latex of the leaves of Aloe Barbadensis Miller (Aloe Vera linné), known in commerce as Curacao Aloe or Aloe Ferox Miller and hybrids of this species, with Aloe Africana Miller and Aloe Spicata Baker, known in commerce as Cape Aloe.

Aloe Vera Oil. The lipid protein obtained from the leaves of Aloe Barbadensis Miller by various solvent extraction processes.

Stabilised Aloe Vera Gel. Synonymous with the term Aloe Vera Gel.

Aloe Vera Pulp. The parenchymal tissue and fibre derived from raw Aloe Vera.

Aloe Vera Concentrate. Aloe Vera Gel, from which natural water has been mechanically removed and which would have a value of 1,500 minimum using the reporting procedure adopted by the NASC.

Reconstituted Aloe Vera Gel. Aloe Vera concentrate, to which an appropriate amount of water has been added to achieve a concentration that is equivalent to 100 per cent Aloe Vera as defined above.

Aloe Vera Gel, Spray Dried. Aqueous derivative of the leaf of Aloe Barbadensis Miller, which has been spray dried on a suitable matrix.

Reconstituted Aloe Vera Gel, Spray Dried. Aloe Vera Gel Spray Dried, to which an appropriatre amount of water has been added to achieve a concentration that is equivalent to 100% Aloe Vera as defined above.

Aloe Vera Gel, Freeze Dried. Aloe Vera Gel that has been freeze dried with or without a matrix.

Reconstituted Aloe Vera Gel, Freeze Dried. Aloe Vera Gel Freeze Dried, to which an appropriate amount of water has been added to achieve a concentration that is equivalent to 100 per cent Aloe Vera as defined above.

Aloe Vera Juice. An ingestible product containing a minimum of 50 per cent Aloe Vera Gel, as defined by the reporting procedure adopted by the NASC.

Aloe Vera Drink. An ingestible product containing less than 50 per cent and more than 10 per cent of aloe vera gel, as defined by the reporting procedure adopted by the NASC.

Aloe Vera Extract. A dilution of Aloe Barbadensis Miller, with water or other suitable solvents that contains less than 10 per cent Aloe Vera, as defined by the reporting procedure adopted by the NASC, and is suitable for ingestion or topical use.

Further reading

Aloe Vera
Carole Miller Kent. Arlington, Virginia
The Print Factory, 1979

Aloe Vera Heals – The Scientific facts
K. Gottlieb. Denver, Colorado
Royal Publications Inc., 1980

The Silent Healer
Bill Coats. 1984

Remarkable Aloe – Aloe Through the Ages
Ivan E. Danhof PhD. M.D.
Omnimedicus Press, 1987

Aloe – Myth Magic Medicine
Odus M Hennessess
Universal Graphics. Lawston O.K. 73502 1990

Aloe Vera The Natural Healer
Paul Hornsey-Pennell
Wordsmith Publishing Company, 1994

Aloe Vera – The Inside Story
Bill Coats 1995

Aloe Vera – Nature's Gift
David Urch
Blackdown Publications, 1999
ISBN 0-9536569-0-X

Aloe Vera – The Health and Healing Plant
Ed Mykut and Marc Schweitzer, 1995

The Essential Aloe Vera
Dr Peter Atherton
Mill Enterprises 2004
ISBN 0-9540896-0-X

Notes

Notes